101 Steps to a Fitter You!

A Common Sense Approach to a Healthier Lifestyle

Evon LaRiese-Davis

iUniverse, Inc.
New York   Bloomington

101 Steps to a Fitter You!
A Common Sense Approach to a Healthier Lifestyle

iUniverse books may be ordered through booksellers or by contacting:

iUniverse
1663 Liberty Drive
Bloomington, IN 47403
www.iuniverse.com
1-800-Authors (1-800-288-4677)

ISBN: 978-1-4401-5317-4 (sc)
ISBN: 978-1-4401-5318-1 (ebk)

Printed in the United States of America

iUniverse rev. date: 8/7/2009

To my Mom, Sedonia M. Davis

At fifteen, I aspired to learning.
At thirty, I established my stand.
At forty, I had no delusions.
At fifty, I knew my destiny.
At sixty, I knew truth in all I heard.
At seventy, I could follow the wishes of my heart without doing wrong.

~ Confucius

CONTENTS

INTRODUCTION

Confessions of a Junk Food Junkie:

When I was in my late 40's, I became more and more aware of how tired I looked (and felt) and how out-of-shape my body had become. Poor eating habits and the lack of physical activity had led to weight gain. Over the years, I had managed to pack on an extra forty pounds of flab. Eat fat not carbs and eat carbs not fat diets, "miracle" belly fat reducing pills, thin thigh machines, flat abs machines—I tried them all. The only thing that shrank was my bank account.

My dining choices in the "old days" read like the perfect storm. Some of the factors that lead up to the catastrophe (my ever-expanding waistline) were:

Breakfast

Hot cakes with extra sausage, bacon, eggs and cheese on a bagel, French toast with extra bacon, or some other "filling" food item was among my daily breakfast preferences. Potato chips and corn chips were not off limits. Moreover, no matter what food item I chose for breakfast, a sixteen-ounce cola always accompanied it.

Snacks

Potato chips, corn chips, and nacho chips were the snacks of choice and I enjoyed them throughout the day.

Lunch

Fried shrimp, a double cheeseburger, a cheese steak, a corned beef sandwich topped with cole slaw, or some other heart attack on a roll accompanied by French fries was the preferred lunch food.

Dinner

Since I disliked cooking, dinner was always a take-out meal. My dinner selections would range from a whole pizza (with lots of toppings) to a cheese steak with extra meat to a full rack of barbecued spare ribs.

The word "extra" was always on the tip of my tongue. I casually outgrew my size eight suits and eventually ate my way to a size fourteen. It was not until the size fourteen pants started to get tight that I had to admit that I was in trouble. I refused to wear a size 16! My first thought was to eat less food at lunchtime. I later decided to take walks at lunchtime instead of eating. Neither of these tactics fostered weight loss. In fact, my weight might have even increased. There were two main reasons my attempts at weight loss had failed. First, I did not change any of my other habits. Secondly, because I did not eat a proper lunch, I was starving later in the afternoon. I would then squelch the sound of my growling stomach by eating unhealthy snacks, i.e., more cola, potato chips, and corn chips.

When I started building my first business, I replaced my fat-laden dinners with evening networking events. Aside from crudités, usually accompanied by high fat dipping sauces, the food and drink served at these events were seldom healthy.

Then, one day I said, "No more!" I decided to grab the flab by the love handles and embark upon a quest to regain control of my body. I searched the web, read health and fitness literature and slowly began to modify my diet and develop an exercise plan. Eating a balanced diet and participating in regular physical activity became the key components of my quest towards a healthier body.

As of this writing, I have dropped two sizes (yes, only two sizes and not a size fourteen to size four in a few months, as seen on TV) and I am on my way to dropping a third size. I feel better and I know that I look better. My goal has never been to wear a size two or even a size four. My goal has been, and will continue to be, to wear a size healthy.

I am not a nutritionist or clinician. I am an everyday woman, just like you, who has decided to reclaim her body. I have had my weight highs and had my weight lows. However, I do not believe in fad dieting. Fad diets or crash diets may have worked for some of you, but they are not diets that most women can maintain for life. I love good food and drink, and cannot ever imagine denying myself something that I enjoy. Therefore, you may see me in a restaurant indulging in a steak, eating eggs with a side of bacon, or sipping a very dry martini. My key to healthy eating is "all things in moderation." I do not drink martinis every evening. I do not eat steaks every night. Moreover, as much as I love bacon, I do not eat bacon every day. Nevertheless, these are things that I enjoy and things in which I indulge from time to time. Keep in mind, I would never go against my doctor's advice and indulge in these extravagances if she ever placed them on my "do not eat" list.

Weight management is a lifelong journey. By taking the time to read "*101 Steps to a Fitter You!*" you have begun your journey towards a healthier lifestyle. So, come on! Let's get started!

PART I

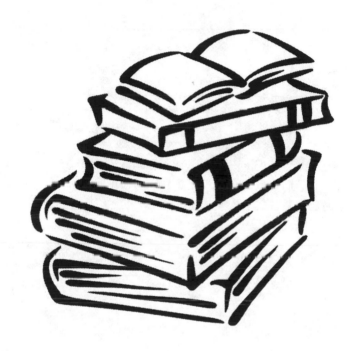

JUST THE FACTS
MA'AM

CHAPTER 1: THE STATISTICS

Stroke is the third leading cause of death and a leading cause of disability; more than 60 percent of all stroke deaths are in women.

~ Journal of the American Heart Association

More than 60 percent of American women are overweight or obese, ensuring that they will neither live well nor live as long as they could.[1] An *overweight* woman has an excess amount of body weight for height. The excess weight can be in the form of muscle, bone, fat and/or body water.[2] An *obese* woman, on the other hand, has an excess accumulation of body fat. Typically, women with 30 percent or more body fat are considered obese.[3] A woman can be overweight without being obese, as in the case of an athlete. Yet, many overweight people are also obese. And, according to a Harvard School of Public Health study,[4] how much you weigh (in relation to your height), your waist size, and how much weight you've gained since your mid-twenties may affect your overall quality of life and may strongly influence your chances of dying early, or having or developing:

- A heart attack, stroke or other cardiovascular disease
- Arthritis
- Diabetes
- Gallstones
- Snoring or sleep apnea
- Cancer of the colon, kidney, breast, or a host of other illnesses

The risks of developing these health issues are even greater for minority women. Health problems such as obesity, diabetes, and hypertension occur more frequently among minority women than with White women.[5] A recent study found that 30 percent of White women were obese, compared with 51 percent of African-American women. Native American women who lived in urban areas had the highest percentage of obese women (63 percent). Forty percent of Mexican-American women were obese—the highest rate among all Latin American/Hispanic women. In stark contrast, Asian American women had the lowest obesity rates among all women. In the Asian American group, Chinese-American women had the lowest obesity rate; only 13.1 percent of Chinese American women were obese.[6]

Physical inactivity is a key element in weight gain. This same study concluded that half of all women over 40 were sedentary. The most sedentary of all were African American women who lived in rural areas; 60 percent of these women led sedentary lifestyles.[7]

Although no one factor is the reason, the four leading causes of death for women[8], in order of prevalence, are:

- Women, overall, and White women: heart disease, cancer, stroke, chronic obstructive pulmonary disease (COPD)
- African-American and Hispanic women: heart disease, cancer, stroke, and diabetes
- American Indian/Alaska native women: heart disease, cancer, unintentional injuries, diabetes
- Asian American/Pacific Islander women: cancer, heart disease, stroke, and diabetes

You might wonder how you can avoid becoming a statistic. Is the deck stacked against you? Absolutely not!

Incorporate some of the suggestions in this book into your daily routine and work with your doctor or other clinician to develop a program that is right for you. Healthy eating, exercise *and* lifestyle modification are the keys to a healthier, longer life.

CHAPTER 2: READING IS FUNDAMENTAL

There is no magic bullet. If you wish to live a better life, you must find time for reading.

The ability to read and understand food labels will become your biggest asset in the battle to attain *and* maintain a fit body. There are three places to look for clues to what is in the food: the Nutrition Facts label, the ingredients list, and the front label of the package.

1. READ THE NUTRITION FACTS LABEL

The Nutrition Facts label is where you will find the Percent Daily Value (% DV) and the daily intake of selected vitamins and nutrients. The Percent Daily Value, as displayed on the Nutrition Facts label, shows the percentage of your total daily intake of nutrients and vitamins contained in one serving of food.

Table 1. Sample Nutrition Facts Label

Nutrition Facts	
Serving Size 1/2 cup (120 mL)	
Servings per Container 2.5	

Amount per Serving	
Calories 70	Calories from Fat 15
	% Daily Value
Total Fat 1.5g	2%
Saturated Fat 0.5g	3%
Trans Fat 0g	
Cholesterol 5mg	2%
Sodium 820mg	34%
Total Carbohydrate 13g	4%
Dietary Fiber 1g	4%
Sugars 1g	
Protein 2g	
Vitamin A	15%
Vitamin C	0%
Calcium	0%
Iron	0%

g = grams   mg = milligrams   mL - milliliters

The bottom portion of the Nutrition Facts label (the footnote) contains the recommended daily limits of fat, cholesterol, and sodium and the recommended daily intake of nutrients such as potassium, carbohydrates and fiber, based on a 2,000 and 2,500 calorie a day diet.

Table 2. Daily Intake/Limit of Selected Nutrients			
Nutrient	Calories	2,000	2,500
Total Fat	Less than	65g	80g
Sat Fat	Less than	20g	25g
Cholesterol	Less than	300mg	300mg
Sodium	Less than	2,400mg	2,400mg
Potassium		3,500mg	3,500mg
Total Carbohydrate		300g	375g
Dietary Fiber		25g	30g

Most of the examples cited in this book are consistent with the 2,000 calorie per day base diet used on the Nutrition Facts Label.

2. USE THE FIVE AND TWENTY RULE

Understanding the Percent Daily Value is easier than you might think. Use the "Five and Twenty" rule: 5 percent is low and 20 percent is high.

Five percent or less is low for all nutrients, for nutrients that should be limited (such as fat, sodium, and cholesterol) and for nutrients that can be consumed in greater quantities (such as fiber, protein, and calcium).[1] Twenty percent or more is high for all nutrients. Remember to look at the serving size. A product label may list the fat DV as 5 percent per serving. However, if the package contains three servings and you consume the entire package, the fat intake becomes 15 percent of the recommended daily limit rather than 5 percent.

3. CHECK THE INGREDIENT LIST

In addition to reading the Nutrition Facts label, you should also look at the *ingredient list*. The Nutrition Facts label shows total sugars, which include both naturally occurring sugars (like those in fruit) as well as those added to the food or drink.[2] The ingredient list is where you are able to determine if the product includes **added** sugars.[3]

When reading the ingredient list, remember that the ingredients are listed in descending order of weight (from most to least).[4] Sugars should not be listed as the first few ingredients. If they are, think of the dietary tradeoffs (Step 13, *Use Dietary Trade-offs*) that you will need to make throughout the rest of the day. Added sugars can appear in the ingredient list as:

5

- Corn syrup
- Lactose
- Maltose
- Dextrose
- Sucrose
- Malt
- Maple sugar
- Brown sugar
- Honey
- Maple syrup
- Sugar
- Light corn syrup
- Dark corn syrup
- Fructose syrup
- Fructose
- Sorghum
- Molasses
- Brown rice syrup
- Powdered sugar
- Glucose
- Concentrated cane syrup
- Fruit juice concentrate
- High fructose corn syrup

The ingredient list also shows artificial sweeteners. Popular artificial sweeteners include *aspartame*, the sweetening ingredient in Equal® and NutraSweet®, and *sucralose*, the sweetening ingredient in Splenda®.

Added fats can appear on a label in a variety of ways. Some examples include hydrogenated oil, partially hydrogenated oil, vegetable oil, corn oil, safflower oil, and palm kernel oil.[5]

SALES PITCH LABELING: CONFUSING CLAIMS

The front of the package is where the sales pitch is located, for example "low fat", "fat free", "whole grain", "natural", "organic", etc. The U.S. Food and Drug Administration has established definitions for the following terms: low, reduced, free, lean, extra lean, and light. So, when these terms are on product packaging, you can feel comfortable knowing that the manufacturers had to be truthful, based upon government standards.[6] Yet, distinguishing the difference between some of these terms can be confusing.

4. GET THE LOW DOWN ON FAT LABELING

Low-fat, reduced fat or fat-free—what is the difference? Items can carry these labels if they meet the following criteria[7]:

> *Low-fat* foods can have no more than 3 grams of fat per serving. You may also think of low-fat foods that are naturally low in fat such as fruits, vegetables, whole grains, and lean proteins.

Fat-free products must contain less than 0.5 grams of fat per serving. Skim milk is an example of a fat-free product.

Reduced fat simply means that the product has less fat than its full-fat version.

However, just because a product label includes these terms does not necessarily mean that the product has fewer calories. Reduced fat and fat-free foods may still be high in sugar or other undesirable nutrients.[8] Using one serving (one-half cup) of vanilla ice cream as an example, Table 3 shows that there is very little difference in the sugar content of these products. In addition, the light ice cream actually contains more sodium than the full-fat version.

Table 3. Nutrient Comparison for One Serving of Ice Cream

	Calories	Calories from Fat	Sodium (mg)	Sugar (g)
Light Creamy Vanilla	100	30	55	13
Fat free Creamy Vanilla	90	0	50	12
Vanilla (full-fat version)	130	60	35	14

Source: Unilever Ice Cream, www.icecreamusa.com

Some snacks, such as potato chips, also use the reduced claim. A one-ounce serving of full-fat potato chips can contain 160 calories and 2.5 grams of saturated fat (12% DV). The reduced fat counterpart may still have as many as 135 calories and 1.5 grams of saturated fat (7% DV) per serving.[9] Table 4 compares the calorie count of some additional reduced fat products with their full-fat counterparts.

Table 4. Fat-Free/Reduced Fat vs. Regular Fat Content

Fat-Free or Reduced Fat	Calories	Regular	Calories
2 tbsp. reduced-fat peanut butter	187	2 tbsp. regular peanut butter	191
3 reduced-fat chocolate chip cookies	118	3 regular chocolate chip cookies	142
2 fat free fig cookies	102	2 regular fig cookies	111
½ c. nonfat vanilla frozen yogurt (<1% fat)	100	½ c. regular whole milk vanilla frozen yogurt (3-4% fat)	104
2 tbsp. fat free caramel topping	103	2 tbsp. caramel topping, homemade with butter	103
½ c. low fat granola cereal	213	½ c. regular granola cereal	257
1 small low fat blueberry muffin	131	1 small regular blueberry muffin	138
1 oz. baked tortilla chips	113	1 oz. regular tortilla chips	143
1 low fat cereal bar (1.3 oz.)	130	1 regular cereal bar (1.3 oz.)	140

Source: U. S. Department of Health and Human Services, National Heart, Lung and Blood Institute

In most cases, the number of calories saved by eating the reduced fat or fat-free product is minimal. Always limit the number and size of portions, even if they are labeled as reduced fat or fat-free.

5. Lighten the Load

Light, when referring to calories and fat, is described as follows: The product contains one-third fewer calories or half the fat of the original product.[10] The term "light" may also be used to describe food in which the sodium content has been reduced by at least 50 percent.[11]

Yogurt with reduced fat content and soup with reduced sodium content are two examples of foods that can carry the label "light".

6. Understand the Difference between "Natural" and "Healthy"

The terms "natural" and "healthy" might also cause confusion. An item that has the term "natural" on its label is always a healthy choice—or is it?

The Food and Drug Administration sets the policy for the use of the term *natural*. Natural simply means the product does not contain synthetic or artificial ingredients.[12] *Healthy,* also defined by government regulation, means the product must meet certain criteria that limit the amounts of fat, saturated fat, cholesterol, and sodium, and require specific minimum amounts of vitamins, minerals, or other beneficial nutrients.[13]

A popular brand of kettle cooked potato chips carries the "All Natural" label.[14] Does this label make potato chips a healthy choice? A one-ounce serving of these chips contains 160 calories and 10 grams of fat. But, how often do you eat only one ounce of potato chips? More often than not, you probably eat the entire 2.5-ounce, 400-calorie, 25 grams of fat bag of potato chips.

7. Choose Organic

Food labeled *organic* must also meet standards set by the government. However, organic food only differs from conventional food in the way it is grown or produced. Organic foods, typically are grown without the use of prohibited pesticides/fertilizers and are free from contamination by human or industrial waste.[15] Organically raised livestock cannot be given antibiotics or hormones to promote.[16]

Eating organic fruits and vegetables can have a major health benefit: Organic foods have less pesticide residue than traditionally grown foods. The non-profit Environmental Working Group (EWG) compiled a list of the forty-five most commonly eaten fruits and vegetables and their pesticide loads, from most contaminated (number 1) to least contaminated (number 45).[17]

Table 5. Pesticide Load Ranked from Worst to Least
for Commonly Eaten Fruits and Vegetables

1. Peaches	16. Cucumbers	31. Watermelon
2. Apples	17. Raspberries	32. Blueberries
3. Sweet bell peppers	18. Plums	33. Papaya
4. Celery	19. Oranges	34. Eggplant
5. Nectarines	20. Grapes (domestic)	35. Broccoli
6. Strawberries	21. Cauliflower	36. Cabbage
7. Cherries	22. Tangerine	37. Bananas
8. Lettuce	23. Mushrooms	38. Kiwi
9. Grapes imported)	24. Cantaloupe	39. Asparagus
10. Pears	25. Lemon	40. Sweet peas (frozen)
11. Spinach	26. Honeydew melon	41. Mango
12. Potatoes	27. Grapefruit	42. Pineapples
13. Carrots	28. Winter squash	43. Sweet corn (frozen)
14. Green beans	29. Tomatoes	44. Avocado
15. Hot peppers	30. Sweet potatoes	45. Onions

Source: The Environmental Working Group, www.foodnews.org

The EWG concluded that people could lower their pesticide exposure by almost 90 percent by avoiding the twelve most contaminated fruits and vegetables on the list and eating the least contaminated

8. BUY LEAN

The term *lean* is something that we frequently see on packaged products. Technically, meat, poultry, and seafood are lean when they contain less than 10 grams of fat and 4.5 grams or less of saturated fat.[18]

Extra lean products contain less than 5 grams of fat and less than 2 grams of saturated fat per serving.[19] Regular ground beef is typically 25 percent fat.[20] A three ounce portion of regular ground beef can contain 236 calories and 6.1 grams of saturated fat. A similar portion of extra lean ground beef might contain only 148 calories and 2.6 grams of saturated fat.[21]

PART 2

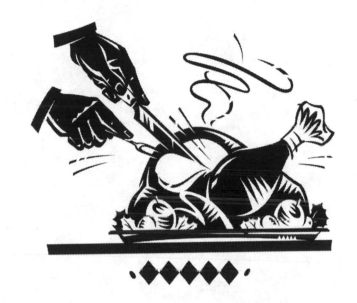

EAT GREAT AND STILL LOSE WEIGHT

CHAPTER 3: GO BACK TO BASICS

If you eat 100 more calories a day than you burn, you will gain about one pound in a month or 10 pounds in a year!

~Health Connections at University Hospital, SUNY

How many of you or your friends have eaten 100 calorie snacks, have been on fat free diets and have avoided carbohydrates like the plague? Eating right and being active can help you maintain or reach a healthy weight. By understanding the role that calories, fats and carbohydrates play in your diet you will be able to enjoy food without fearing these words and make decisions that contribute to a healthier body and a happier life.

Calories provide a measure of how much energy you get from your food. Fats and carbohydrates give you that energy. The problem with calories is that many women consume more calories than they need. You should be aware that, no matter how good the carbohydrate and how much better the fat, if you do not expend that energy, it all ends up as unwanted pounds. Therefore, it might be time to go back to the basics: eat fresh and simple.

9. BREAK THE FAST

Breakfast is the most important meal of the day. Your body has been in a state of fasting since you went to bed the night before and it now needs energy to help you function throughout the rest of the day. Breakfast helps to provide that energy. One study found that breakfast eaters have one-half the risk of developing obesity and insulin resistance, a major risk factor for diabetes and heart disease, compared with breakfast skippers.[1]

Breakfast should include a combination of foods from the four major food groups: milk, meat, fruits and vegetables, and grains. However, being on the go, we oftentimes grab whatever happens to be convenient. Look at four popular breakfast choices:

"Food . . . Fast"

A breakfast sandwich comprised of one 4.8-ounce egg, Canadian-style bacon, and American cheese on an English muffin: three hundred calories, 110 calories from fat, twelve grams of fat, five grams of saturated fat, 820 milligrams of sodium, and three grams of sugars[2]

"The Java Jolt"

A twenty-ounce espresso with steamed whole milk and topped with foam: 290 calories, 140 calories from fat, 15 grams of fat, 9 grams of saturated fat, 190 milligrams of sodium, 21 grams of sugars[3]

"Little Miss Muffin"

One apple-bran muffin: 310 calories, 60 calories from fat, 7 grams of fat, 2 grams of saturated fat, 440 milligrams of sodium, 29 grams of sugars[4]

"Stoned Scone"

One blueberry scone: 480 calories, 180 calories from fat, 21 grams of fat, 8 grams of saturated fat, 350 milligrams of sodium, 16 grams of sugars[5]

Based on a 2,000 calorie a day diet, the dietary guidelines established by the U.S. Department of Agriculture limit fat calories to 20 to 35% of total calories, saturated fat to 20 grams or less, cholesterol to less than 300 mg, and sodium to less than 2400 mg.[6] The scone contains nearly one-quarter of your daily calorie needs; the breakfast sandwich contains more than one-third of your total daily maximum of sodium! The espresso contains nearly as many fat calories as the breakfast sandwich and the muffin combined!

You may choose to exclude all of these items from your breakfast selection unless you are willing to make some modifications to the meals that you eat throughout the rest of the day. Some better breakfast options might include:

- Low-fat yogurt sprinkled with low-fat granola
- Oatmeal with low-fat, fat-free milk, or soy milk
- A slice of whole-wheat toast with a thin spread of peanut butter
- A fruit smoothie made with frozen fruit, low-fat yogurt, and juice
- High-fiber, low-sugar cereal with soy milk or low-fat milk

10. EAT MORE TO LOSE WEIGHT

Eat five to six meals a day. This might sound like you will eat a lot of food. Yet, eating five to six *small* meals throughout the course of the day can be beneficial. When you are at the office, you may find yourself thinking, "I can hardly wait until it's time for dinner. I'm starving!" Then, you grab an unhealthy snack or, when you get home, you just pig out!

Enjoy a small, healthy snack between breakfast and lunch, and eat another healthy snack between lunch and dinner. Doing this may help you feel fuller throughout the day, making you less likely to overeat at either meal. Eating a light snack after dinner may help you feel less hungry when you get up in the morning.

Choose snacks from different food groups. Eat a handful of almonds or pair some apple slices, a couple of small multi-grain pretzels, or a couple of banana slices with a dab of chunky peanut butter. If you eat smart at other meals, potato chips or some chocolate can be occasional snacks. Try substituting some of the options listed in Table 6 for your usual snacks:

Table 6. Snack Options

Instead of . . .	Substitute . . .	Calories Saved
Oil-popped popcorn (3 cups)	Air-popped popcorn (3 cups)	73
Six peanut butter crackers from the vending machine	An 8 oz. container of no sugar added non fat yogurt	82
Sweetened drinks	Sparkling water	136
Three chocolate sandwich cookies	One large orange	54

Source: "Healthy Eating for Healthy Weight: Cutting Calories", Centers for Disease Control and Prevention

11. BEWARE OF LOCAL TRADITIONS

While researching data for this book, I came across a study about the Philadelphia cheese steak. Dietitians from the University of Pennsylvania Health System[7] conducted the study.

A "Philly" cheese steak typically consists of very thinly sliced steak meat, melted cheese, and onions served on a long roll. A side of cheese fries often accompanies the cheese steak. Cheese fries are nothing more than French fries topped with melted cheese. The dietitians visited some cheese steak eateries and came up with the following analysis of these Philadelphia (Pennsylvania) favorites: the cheese steak contained 900 calories and 40 grams of fat; the cheese fries contained 870 calories and 50 grams of fat. When you visit Philadelphia, split the cheese steak with a friend, skip the fries and save 1,320 calories and 70 grams of fat!

12. COMPARE LABELS

Serving sizes are generally consistent for similar types of foods.[8] Look at the serving size and then use the %DV on the Nutrition Facts labels to easily identify which products are higher or lower in certain nutrients. You can also use the %DV to help you quickly distinguish one claim from another, such as "reduced fat" and "light." Just compare the %DV in each food product to see which one is higher or lower in that nutrient.

13. USE DIETARY TRADE-OFFS

You do not always have to give up a favorite food to eat a healthy diet. When a food you like is high in fat, balance it by eating lower fat foods at other times of the day. Use the %DV listed on the Nutrition Facts label to help you make dietary trade-offs.[9] Pay attention to how much fat you eat so that the **total** amount of fat for the day stays below 100%DV. For example, if your lunchtime selection is the high calorie Philly cheese steak (Step 11, *Beware of Local Traditions*), then choose a salad with a lean protein for dinner.

14. DRINK PLENTY OF WATER

Recent studies have expressed differing views about the appropriate amount of water that one should drink. I will not debate the merits of these studies. We all know that proper hydration is necessary to maintain a healthy body. A University of Utah study found that eight 8-ounce glasses of water a day "helps maintain the body's hydration status."[10] Eating foods with high water content, such as fruits and vegetables, can also contribute to your fluid goal.[11] Water is sugar-free and calorie-free. Substitute water for calorie-based drinks.

15. LIMIT YOUR INTAKE OF SOFT DRINKS

Consider the following: An eight-ounce can of cola may contain as many as 100 calories, 28 grams of sugar, and 20 mg of sodium.[12] Soda contains empty calories, i.e., calories with little or no nutritional value.

You may opt to drink zero-calorie beverages. These drinks usually contain artificial sweeteners such as aspartame and sucralose. To use artificial sweeteners or not to use them is a personal choice. The prospect of drinking a cola or other drink that tastes sweet and has zero calories might sound thrilling. However, drinking zero-calorie drinks may have unexpected side effects.

A University of Texas study suggested that people who drink diet sodas might have a greater chance of becoming overweight or obese. Researchers concluded that this may be due to a person not changing the rest of her lifestyle.[13] You may also find yourself eating more food than you would normally eat because you feel secure in the knowledge that you saved calories with the zero-calorie soft drink.

16. USE CAUTION WITH FLAVORED AND VITAMIN-INFUSED WATERS

Water does not have any calories. But a bottle of flavored or vitamin infused water can be loaded with as many, if not more, calories than a can of soda. The Nutrition Facts label on a popular brand of vitamin water lists 50 calories and 13 grams of sugar per serving. The serving size is 8 ounces. However, the bottle contains 20 ounces or 2.5 servings.[14] Stick to the serving size if you are watching your calorie count.

17. Go Lean with Protein

There are two main sources of protein: animals and plants. Protein is essential to the growth and repair of muscle tissue. Protein might also aid in weight loss for the following reasons[15]:

- High-protein foods slow the movement of food from your stomach to your intestine. As a result, you may feel fuller longer.
- Protein does not cause the same rise in blood sugar and increase in hunger as the blood sugar falls, such as that which occurs when you eat carbohydrates such as white bread.
- Your body uses more energy to digest protein than it does to digest fats or carbohydrates.

Lean protein such as meat and poultry should be among the staples of your new eating style. However, when choosing protein-rich foods, be aware of other things that come along with the protein such as fat and saturated fat. Include lean cuts of beef such as flank, skinless chicken and turkey breasts, and lean ground turkey (no more than 8% fat).[16] Limit your intake of fattier meat products such as chuck or blade roast, regular ground beef, bacon, and poultry with the skin intact.

18. Look for Dairy and Plant Protein

Dairy products are good sources of protein. Include products such as low-fat cottage cheese, ricotta, and yogurt in your meals. The Nutrition Facts label will help you determine the protein content of these products.

Legumes, nuts, and whole grains not only supply protein, but also contain fiber, vitamins, and minerals. Incorporate soybeans, couscous, pinto beans, red kidney beans, and chickpeas (garbanzo beans), among others, into your daily diet.[17]

19. Get Two to Three Servings of Protein a Day

Two to three servings of protein-rich foods will meet the needs of most healthy adults. Recommended serving sizes for protein include[18]:

- 2 to 3 ounces of cooked lean meat, poultry, or fish (a portion about the size of a deck of playing cards)

- 1/2 cup of cooked dried beans
- 1 egg, 2 tablespoons of peanut butter, or 1 ounce of cheese

CHAPTER 4: EAT FRESH

Research shows that if you eat a low-calorie appetizer before a meal, you will eat fewer total calories during the meal. Start your meals with a broth-based soup or a green salad without a large amount of cheese, or croutons.

~Centers for Disease Control and Prevention

In order to lose weight, you must eat fewer calories than your body uses. Eating fruits and vegetables can help you reach that goal. Most fruits and vegetables are low in fats and calories. An added bonus is that the water and fiber in fruits and vegetables may help you fell fuller. Eating fruits and vegetables may also reduce the risk of some cancers and chronic diseases.[1]

20. FOCUS ON FRUITS

Fruits are a good source of fiber, vitamins, and nutrients. Choose fresh or frozen fruits over canned fruit or juices. Canned fruits and commercial juices may contain unwanted added sugars and lack the fiber that you will get by eating fresh fruits. If fresh fruits are not available, you can also substitute dried fruit. Dried fruits contain the same vitamins, minerals, and antioxidants as fresh fruits but, cup for cup, may contain more calories. For example, a small box of raisins contains 100 calories as compared to an entire cup of grapes, which also contains 100 calories.[2] To avoid excess calories when eating dried fruits, choose those that are unsweetened or sweetened with 100% fruit juice and limit the portion size.

Fresh fruits are an excellent source of Vitamin A and Vitamin C. Vitamin A plays an important role in regulating your immune system.[3] A healthy immune system helps prevent or fight off infections. Vitamin A also helps to keep the eyes and skin healthy.[4] Fruits that supply Vitamin A include cantaloupe, apricots, papaya, mango, oranges, and peaches.[5] Vitamin C helps heal cuts and wounds and keep teeth and gums healthy.[6] Citrus fruits, such as oranges, contain Vitamin C.

The amount of fruit you need to eat depends upon your age, sex, and level of physical activity. Women 40 years of age and older who get less than 30 minutes of moderate physical activity a day should eat at least one and one-half cups of fruit each day.[7] More active women may be able to eat more.

Table 7. Fruit Servings

Fruit	Amount that counts as 1 cup
Apple	½ large (3.25" diameter) or 1 small (2.5" diam.)
Applesauce	1 cup
Banana	1 large (8" to 9" long)
Cantaloupe	1 cup diced or melon balls
Grapes	32 seedless grapes
Grapefruit	1 medium (4" diameter)
Mixed fruit (fruit cocktail)	1 cup
Orange	1 large (3-1/16" diameter)
Orange, mandarin	1 cup canned, drained
Peach	1 large (2 ¾" diameter) or 2 halves, canned
Pear	1 medium pear (2.5 per lb)
Pineapple	1 cup
Plum	3 medium or 2 large plums
Strawberries	About 8 large berries
Watermelon	1 small wedge (1" thick)
Dried fruit	½ cup dried fruit
100% fruit juice	1 cup

Source: U.S. Department of Agriculture, MyPyramid.gov

21. VARY YOUR VEGETABLES

Eat fresh, colorful vegetables. Colorful vegetables are great sources of potassium, Vitamin E and, just as with fresh fruits, Vitamins A and C.[8] Diets rich in potassium may help to maintain a healthy blood pressure[9] while Vitamin E helps protect Vitamin A and essential fatty acids from cell oxidation.[10] The USDA divides vegetables into five subgroups, based on their nutrient content[11]:

> **Dark green vegetables** such as bok choy, broccoli, collard greens, dark green leafy lettuce, kale, mesclun, mustard greens, romaine lettuce, spinach, turnip greens, and watercress

Orange vegetables such as acorn squash, butternut squash, carrots, hubbard squash, pumpkin, and sweet potatoes

Dry beans and peas, including black beans, black-eyed peas, garbanzo beans (chickpeas), kidney beans, lentils, lima beans (mature), navy beans, pinto beans, soy beans, split peas, tofu (bean curd made from soybeans), and white beans

Starchy vegetables like corn, green peas, lima beans (green), and potatoes

Other vegetables, including artichokes, asparagus, bean sprouts, cabbage, cauliflower, celery, cucumbers, eggplant, green beans, green or red peppers, iceberg lettuce, mushrooms, okra, onions, parsnips, tomatoes, tomato juice, vegetable juice, turnips, wax beans, and zucchini

Sweet potatoes, white potatoes, white beans, lima beans, cooked greens, and carrot juice provide potassium.[12] You get Vitamin E when you eat green vegetables such as spinach and broccoli. Pumpkin, carrots, spinach beans, sweet potatoes, turnip greens, mustard greens, kale, collard greens, and red peppers supply Vitamin A.[13] Vegetables rich in Vitamin C include red and green peppers, sweet potatoes, kale, broccoli, and cauliflower.[14]

22. CUT CALORIES BY EATING FRUITS AND VEGETABLES

Substitute the high-calories ingredients in some of your favorite dishes with low-calorie fruits and vegetables. The water and fiber in fruits and vegetables will add volume to your dishes, allowing you to eat the same amount of food with fewer calories.

Choose fruits and vegetables for your snacks and enjoy 100-calorie snacks without the words that you cannot pronounce in the ingredient list and the added sugars and fats.[15]

- A medium-size apple - 72 calories
- A medium-size banana - 105 calories
- One cup steamed green beans - 44 calories
- One cup blueberries - 83 calories
- One cup grapes - 100 calories
- One cup carrots - 45 calories
- One cup broccoli - 30 calories
- One cup bell peppers with 2 tbsp. hummus - 46 calories

CHAPTER 5: EAT CALCIUM-RICH FOODS

Women are four times more likely than men to get osteoporosis and comprise eighty percent of those affected by this disease.

~National Osteoporosis Foundation

Osteoporosis is a disease in which the bones become fragile and are likely to break. Calcium helps to maintain strong bones. Although the majority of the calcium in your body is found in your bones and teeth, your body cannot create calcium on its own.[1] When your body does not get enough calcium through food, calcium is taken from your bones. You need to eat the right foods to help replace the calcium that is lost on a daily basis through your skin, hair, nails, feces, sweat, and urine.[2]

23. KNOW YOUR NUMBERS

The Nutrition Facts Label lists calcium as a percentage of the DV. This percentage is based on one thousand milligrams of calcium per day. For example, 30 %DV of calcium equals 300 milligrams of calcium; 15% DV of calcium equals 150 milligrams of calcium.[3]

Women under 50 should get at least 1,000 milligrams of calcium and 400-800 IU of vitamin D daily, and women over 50 should get at least 1,200 milligrams of calcium and 800-1,000 IU of vitamin D daily. Your body needs Vitamin D for optimal calcium absorption. Limit your total daily calcium intake from all sources to no more than 2,000 - 2,500 milligrams.[4]

24. UNDERSTAND THE CALCIUM CLAIMS

Many food packages include a claim such as "High in Calcium." Use the following as a guide to help understand the calcium claims[5] on food labels:

"High in Calcium," "Rich in Calcium," or an "Excellent Source of Calcium": The food contains twenty percent or more of the calcium DV.

"Contains Calcium," "Provides Calcium," or is a "Good Source of Calcium": The food contains ten to nineteen percent of the calcium DV.

"Calcium Enriched," "Calcium-Fortified," or has "More Calcium": The food contains ten percent or more of the calcium DV, when compared to a standard serving size of a similar food.

25. Choose Three Servings of Dairy Each Day

Dairy products are high in calcium and can easily provide more than one-third of your daily calcium needs. It is easy to eat the recommended three servings a day[6], by choosing products such as yogurt, cheese, and milk.

Table 8. Calcium Content of Dairy Products

	Serving Size	Calcium Content (mg)
Plain nonfat yogurt	8 oz.	415
Plain low-fat yogurt	8 oz.	415
Swiss cheese	1.5 oz.	408
Chocolate milk shake	10 oz.	374
Mozzarella cheese (part skim)	1.5 oz.	311
Cheddar cheese	1.5 oz.	306
Fruit-flavored low fat yogurt	8 oz.	345
Skim milk	1 cup	316
1% low fat milk	1 cup	313
2% reduced fat milk	1 cup	297
Whole milk	1 cup	291
1% low fat chocolate milk	1 cup	287
2% reduced fat chocolate milk	1 cup	284
Chocolate milk	1 cup	280

National Dairy Council, www.nebmilk.org

26. Purchase Calcium-Fortified Foods

Fortified food is a food to which a nutrient, not already present in the food, is added for health purposes. Examples of calcium-fortified foods are orange juice and cereal. Check the product label to determine the calcium content. For example, a box of calcium-fortified corn flakes may include the following statement: "Calcium Enriched (fifteen percent more of the Daily Value than non-fortified corn flakes)."

27. EAT NON-DAIRY FOODS THAT NATURALLY CONTAIN CALCIUM

Calcium occurs naturally in many non-dairy foods such as green vegetables, fruits, seafood, and nuts.

Table 9. Calcium Content of Non-Dairy Foods

	Serving Size	Calcium Content
Sardines with bones	3 oz.	371mg
Canned pink salmon with bones	3 oz.	181mg
Almonds, dried, roasted, whole	1/3 c.	126mg
English muffin, enriched	1	98mg
Kale, frozen cooked	½ c.	90mg
Okra, frozen cooked	½ c.	88mg
Beet greens, fresh cooked	½ c.	82mg
Orange	1	52mg
Broccoli, fresh cooked, chopped	½ c.	47mg

Source: National Dairy Council

CHAPTER 6: REDUCE SODIUM INTAKE

Most Americans consume between 3,000 and 20,000 mg of sodium a day.
~Healthline/The Gale Group, Inc.[1]

You may be one of the many women who add salt to food before tasting it. When dining out, trust the chef! Her training and experience have taught her how to properly season food. Moreover, depending upon the restaurant and the dish, there may already be more sodium in that meal than you care to ingest.

Sodium is a mineral used to flavor or preserve foods. Salt is a compound of sodium and chloride. Sodium intake should be limited to less than 2400 mg (1 teaspoon of salt) per day. For individuals with hypertension, Blacks, and middle-aged and older adults, the limit is even lower. The National Institutes of Health recommends that members of these groups consume less than 1500 milligrams of sodium per day.[2] The dietary limit includes sodium and salt from all sources including what's already in the product, what is added during cooking and what is added at the table. Increased sodium intake has been linked to an increased risk of developing high blood pressure.[3]

Food manufacturers add many different sodium compounds to foods. When reading the labels, you should look for both salt **and** sodium, including kosher salt and sea salt, as well as the word "soda." Also, check the label for the following sodium compounds[4]:

- *Sodium alginate* - used in many chocolate milks and ice creams to make a smooth mixture
- *Sodium bicarbonate (baking soda)* - used to leaven breads and cakes; sometimes added to vegetables in cooking
- *Sodium benzoate* - used as a preservative in many condiments such as relishes, sauces and salad dressings
- *Sodium hydroxide* - used in food processing to soften and loosen skins of ripe olives and certain fruits and vegetables
- *Sodium nitrite* - used in cured meats and sausages

- *Sodium propionate* - used in pasteurized cheese and in some breads and cakes to inhibit growth of molds
- *Sodium sulfite* - used to bleach certain fruits such as maraschino cherries and glazed or crystallized fruits that are to be artificially colored; also used as a preservative in some dried fruits such as prunes
- *Disodium phosphate* - found in some quick-cooking cereals and processed cheeses
- *Monosodium glutamate (MSG)* - seasoning used in home, restaurant and hotel cooking and in many packaged, canned and frozen foods

28. LIMIT OR AVOID PROCESSED FOODS

You easily reach the maximum daily allowance of 2400 mg of sodium and more when you do not eat the proper foods. Processed foods are a major source of sodium consumed.

Table 10. Sodium Content of Selected Foods

Food	Serving Size	Sodium (mg)
Breads	1 oz.	95-210
Frozen cheese pizza	4 oz.	450-1200
Frozen vegetables	½ c.	2-160
Salad dressing	2 tbsp	110-505
Salsa	2 tbsp.	150-240
Soup (tomato), reconstituted	8 oz.	700-1260
Tomato juice	8 oz. (1 c.)	340-1040
Potato chips	1 oz.	120-180
Tortilla chips	1 oz.	105-160
Pretzels	1 oz.	290-560

Source: Dietary Guidelines for Americans, 2005

Limit or avoid frozen dinners, pizzas, canned soups and broths, salad dressings, smoked, processed or cured beef, poultry and pork. These products all have high sodium content. Make your own pizzas; make oil and vinegar salad dressings. If you must buy canned soups and broths, look for words or phrases such as: sodium free, very low sodium, low sodium, reduced (or less) sodium, light in sodium, and unsalted.

29. USE FRESH HERBS WHEN COOKING

If you think that only salt and pepper give foods flavor, try using less salt and adding fresh herbs. Fresh herbs such as rosemary, flat leaf parsley, cilantro, thyme, garlic and others add flavor as well as variety to foods. When you cannot find fresh herbs, substitute dried herbs, keeping in mind that the dried version is much more potent that the fresh version. Try seasoning your meat, poultry, or fish with some of the following spices and herbs[5]:

- Bay leaf, marjoram, nutmeg, onion, pepper (beef)
- Curry powder, garlic, rosemary, mint (lamb)
- Garlic, onion, sage, pepper, oregano (pork)
- Bay leaf, curry powder, ginger, marjoram (veal)
- Ginger, marjoram, oregano, paprika, poultry seasoning, rosemary, sage, tarragon, thyme (chicken)
- Curry powder, dill, dry mustard, lemon juice, marjoram, paprika, pepper (fish)

Spices and herbs lend flavor to vegetables as well[6]:

- Cumin, curry powder, onion, paprika (corn)
- Cinnamon, cloves, marjoram, nutmeg, rosemary, sage (carrots)
- Dill, curry powder, lemon juice, marjoram, oregano, tarragon, thyme (green beans)
- Ginger, marjoram, onion, parsley, sage (peas)
- Dill, garlic, onion, paprika, parsley, sage (potatoes)
- Cloves, curry powder, marjoram, nutmeg, rosemary, sage (summer squash)
- Cinnamon, ginger, nutmeg, onion (winter squash)
- Basil, bay leaf, dill, marjoram, onion, oregano, parsley, pepper (tomatoes)

30. USE MY "SALT IN THE PALM" METHOD

Typically, people salt their food by violently shaking the salt container until they think a sufficient layer of salt covers the food. Sprinkle the amount of salt that you would normally shake onto food into the palm of your hand. Pour the salt that was in the palm of your hand into a teaspoon. You will be surprised at how much salt you almost added to your meal. Remember, you should limit your sodium intake to no more than the equivalent of 1 teaspoon of salt per day.

CHAPTER 7: EAT MORE CARBOHYDRATES

Eat at least three ounces of whole-grain cereals, breads, crackers, rice, or pasta every day. One ounce is about one slice of bread, one cup of breakfast cereal, or ½ cup of cooked rice or pasta.

~U.S. Office on Women's Health

Carbohydrates are good for you. What an odd statement to make! Or is it? You or some of your friends may be on low carb/no carb diets. You may ask, "How can carbs be good for me?"

Carbohydrates or "carbs" are the preferred source of energy for your body. Your body breaks down carbohydrates into glucose (blood sugar) that your blood carries to your cells to use for energy.[1] Carbohydrates are the sugars and starches found in foods like bread, pasta, cereals, fruits, honey, syrup, vegetables, and table sugar. A carbohydrate is classified as either simple or complex, depending upon how fast your body digests and absorbs the sugars.[2] Simple carbohydrates (also called simple sugars) are found in refined (processed) sugars, such as the white sugar typically found on your tables. Complex carbohydrates, also known as starches and dietary fiber, include grain products such as bread, crackers, pasta, and rice.[3]

31. UNDERSTAND SIMPLE SUGARS

Many foods contain carbohydrates, which are broken down into simple sugars. Not only are simple sugars the refined sugars that you sprinkle onto your cereal but they are also the sugars that serve as the basis of many candies. Simple sugars can also be found naturally in food such as fruit and milk.[4] What is the difference between the refined sugars and the naturally occurring simple sugars? Refined sugars contain empty calories. In contrast, foods with naturally occurring sugars have nutritional value; they contain vitamins and nutrients in addition to the sugars.

32. Make Half Your Grains Whole

Complex carbohydrates, such as grains, are better choices than simple carbohydrates. Any food made from wheat, rice, oats, cornmeal, barley or another cereal grain is a grain product. Grains are either *refined* or *unrefined*. Refined grains, such as white flour have been processed, which removes nutrients and fiber.[5] Unrefined grains, known as whole grains, still contain the vitamins and nutrients and are also rich in fiber.[6] The USDA considers grains as "whole" when nothing has been taken away or added by processing. Grains are contained in a kernel; whole grains contain the entire grain kernel. Whole grains provide fiber, energy and vitamins, and help to promote regularity and possibly decrease risk of heart disease.[7] Check the ingredient list for the words "whole grain" or "whole-wheat" when purchasing products. Some common whole grain products include[8]:

- Brown rice
- Buckwheat
- Bulgur (cracked wheat)
- Oatmeal
- Popcorn
- Whole-wheat cereal flakes
- Muesli
- Whole grain barley

- Whole grain cornmeal
- Whole rye
- Whole-wheat bread
- Whole-wheat crackers
- Whole-wheat pasta
- Whole-wheat sandwich buns
- Whole-wheat tortillas
- Wild rice

Eating foods high in fiber may help reduce cholesterol and help prevent colon cancer.[9] Foods with high fiber content also make you feel fuller so you are less likely to overeat.

33. Monitor Refined Grains Intake

Refined grains have been *milled* or processed. Milling grains gives them a finer texture and longer shelf life than whole grains. The milling process also removes iron, dietary fiber and some B vitamins.[10] Some refined grains are *enriched* to add back iron and certain B vitamins (thiamin, riboflavin, niacin, folic acid) that were removed during processing; fiber is not added back to enriched grains. Look for the word "enriched" in the ingredient list when purchasing refined grains. Some examples of refined grains include[11]:

- Cornbread
- Corn tortillas
- Couscous
- Crackers
- Flour tortillas
- Grits
- Noodles
- Spaghetti

- White flour
- Macaroni
- Pitas
- Pretzels
- Corn flakes
- White bread
- White sandwich buns
- White rice

CHAPTER 8: BECOME FRIENDS WITH FATS

Eat less than 7% of your total calories as saturated fat.
~ The American Diabetics Association

There are four major types of fats that work their way into our diets: saturated fats, trans fats, monounsaturated fats, and polyunsaturated fats.[1] Contrary to what you might believe, fats can be your friends. The key is to distinguish between better fats and worse fats.

Just as with carbohydrates, the body needs fats for energy. Fats also help to protect your organs, keep your body warm, and absorb some nutrients. The problem with fats is that most people eat too much fat or the wrong type of fat.

The first two fats, saturated and trans fats (trans fatty acids), are the fats that are linked to heart disease and other health disorders. The better fats, monounsaturated and polyunsaturated fats, are thought to be beneficial, when eaten in moderation, and may help to lower cholesterol.

34. LIMIT SATURATED AND TRANS FATS

Saturated fats tend to be solid at room temperature, like lard or a stick of butter. Imagine those little fats working their way into your blood stream and solidifying. That is not a pretty picture.

Eating foods high in saturated fats may increase the chance of developing heart disease. Saturated fats occur naturally in many foods and come mainly from animal sources. Foods that contain saturated fats are often also high in cholesterol. Examples of saturated fats or food containing saturated fats[2] include:

- Cheeseburger
- Lamb
- Butter
- Full-fat cheese

- Chocolate
- Coconut oil
- Poultry skin
- Bologna

- Palm oil
- Cream
- Ice cream
- Whole milk
- 2% milk
- Sour cream
- Lard
- Salt pork

- Regular ground beef
- Cream sauces
- Sausage
- Bacon
- Spareribs
- Coconut milk
- Gravy made with meat drippings

Trans fats also tend to be solid at room temperature. Unlike saturated fats, most trans fats you eat are created by an industrial process that adds hydrogen to vegetable oils to make them more solid. *Hydrogenated oil* and *partially hydrogenated oil* are other names for trans fats. Eating trans fats raises your bad cholesterol (LDL), lowers your good cholesterol (HDL), and increases your chances of developing heart disease or stroke.[3] These fats are frequently found in packaged and baked foods. Some trans fats occur naturally in foods such as beef and lamb. It is unknown as to whether naturally occurring trans fat has the same effect as its industrially produced counterpart.[4] Trans fats[5] are found in:

- Donuts
- Biscuits
- French fries
- Shortening
- Pie crusts
- Crackers

- Stick margarine
- Pizza dough
- Potato chips
- Muffins
- Cakes
- Cookies

You should know that just because a product is labeled "trans fat free" does not mean it is healthy. The food could still be loaded with saturated fats or, in some cases, added sugars.

You should also be aware of the content of 90- and 100-calorie foods. Look at the ingredient list of a popular 90-calorie snack:

> Ingredients: Whole grain rolled oats, whole grain puffed cereal (whole grain white corn, whole grain oat flour, whole wheat flour, whole grain brown rice flour, *sugar*, calcium carbonate, *salt*, (BHT (a preservative)), *sugar*, *partially hydrogenated palm kernel and palm oil*, nonfat dry milk, *high fructose corn syrup*, *polydextrose,* soybean oil, dried *whole milk*, soy lecithin, *cocoa, cocoa*

processed with alkali, molasses, honey, sodium bicarbonate, natural and artificial flavors.

Once you get beyond the whole grains, you will find that the product contains added sugars, sodium, and fats, including trans fat laden partially hydrogenated palm kernel and palm oil. What lesson have you learned? Even when a snack is labeled "90-calorie" or "100-calorie", you still need to read the ingredient list. Be aware of what you are eating and adjust your meals accordingly.

35. INCORPORATE MUFAS, PUFAS AND OMEGA-3S INTO YOUR DIET

The better fats, monounsaturated fat and polyunsaturated fat, are high in Vitamin E and might help reduce the risk of heart disease and help stimulate "good cholesterol". Monounsaturated fats (MUFAs) tend to be liquid at room temperature and solid when chilled. Foods containing monounsaturated fats[6] include:

- Canola oil
- Peanuts
- Pecans
- Olive oil
- Olives
- Peanut butter
- Peanut oil
- Avocados
- Almonds
- Sesame seeds
- Sunflower oil
- Cashews

Polyunsaturated fats (PUFAs) are liquid at room temperature and when chilled. Like monounsaturated fats, polyunsaturated fats can help lower cholesterol and reduce the chances of heart disease. Sources of polyunsaturated fats[7] include:

- Salmon
- Herring
- Corn oil
- Pumpkin seeds
- Trout
- Sunflower seeds
- Mackerel
- Safflower oil
- Cottonseed oil
- Walnuts
- Soft (tub) margarine

- Soybean oil

Polyunsaturated fats contain Omega-3 fatty acids. Omega-3 fatty acids help prevent clogging of the arteries.[8] Foods containing Omega-3 fatty acids include:

- Herring
- Mackerel
- Salmon
- Sardines
- Canola oil
- Walnuts
- Flaxseed
- Flaxseed oil
- Rainbow trout
- Tofu

You may not find the amount of MUFAs or PUFAs listed on the Nutrition Facts label. However, you can calculate the amount of unsaturated fat by using the following formula[9]:

Total Fat - (Saturated fat + Trans Fat) = Total monounsaturated and polyunsaturated fats

The following list of oils is from most to least percentage of unsaturated fat[10]:

Canola oil	94%
Safflower oil	90%
Sunflower oil	89%
Corn oil	87%
Olive oil	86%
Soybean oil	85%
Margarine, tub	83%
Peanut oil	82%
Margarine, stick	80%
Cottonseed oil	73%
Solid vegetable shortening	68%
Lard	59%
Palm oil	48%
Butter	34%
Palm kernel oil	13%
Coconut oil	8%

36. Eat at Least Two Servings of Fish per Week

The American Heart Association recommends that you try to eat at least two servings of fish per week, especially fish like salmon, tuna, sardines and mackerel, because they are high in omega-3 fatty acids. Fish such as swordfish, shark, king mackerel, and tilefish should be avoided to minimize your exposure to mercury.[11] Albacore (white) tuna should be limited to one six-ounce serving per week.[12] Albacore tuna has more mercury than canned light tuna.[13] Choose wild salmon over farm-raised, due to concentrated levels of dioxins and PCBs in farm-raised salmon. PCBs and dioxins, which have links to cancer and other issues, can stay in your body for years.[14]

37. Use Moderation, Even When Eating the Better Fats

All fats are high in calories and contain the same number of calories—9 calories per gram. In contrast, carbohydrates and proteins contain only 4 calories per serving.[15] The calories from fat in one serving should be no more than twenty to thirty-five percent of the total calories.[16] If the label does not list the percentage of fat in the food, you can calculate the fat percentage by dividing the number of calories from fat by the number of total calories and multiplying that number by 100:

(Calories from fat/Total calories) x 100 = percent of fat

For example, if a 200-calorie food item has 40 calories from fat, you divide 40 by 200 and then multiply the result by 100:

(40/200) x 100 = 20

The result, 20, means that 20% of the food's calories come from fat.

Based on a 2,000 calorie per day diet, the American Heart Association[17] recommends that the total amount of fat consumed each day is no more than 25-35 percent of your total daily calories. Within these limits, saturated fats consumed should be less than seven percent of the total daily calories and trans fat consumption should be less than one percent. Translating these percentages into numbers:

- approximately 56–78 grams (500–700 of those calories) from fats;
- less than 16 grams (less than 140 of those calories) from saturated fats; and
- less than 2 grams (less than 20 of those calories) from *trans* fats.

38. Know the Difference between HDL and LDL Cholesterol

Cholesterol is a soft, waxy substance found in the bloodstream and in your body's cells. Your body needs cholesterol. Cholesterol is used by your body to produce cell membranes and some hormones and to support other body functions.[18] But, just as eating too many calories can cause problems, having too much of the wrong type of cholesterol in your blood can lead to health issues.

Cholesterol comes from two sources: your body and the food that you eat. Your liver and cells produce about 75 percent of your blood cholesterol. The other 25 percent comes from food.[19] The "good" cholesterol (HDL), is thought to protect against heart disease, possibly by carrying cholesterol away from the arteries and back to the liver, where it is passed through the body.[20]

Foods that are high in saturated fats can raise the LDL or "bad" cholesterol levels.[21] Too much LDL cholesterol can build up in the arteries and form plaque, narrowing the arteries and increasing the risk of a heart attack or stroke.[22] Foods to avoid or limit because of their high cholesterol content[23] include: fatty cuts of beef, lamb and pork, hot dogs, bacon, regular ground beef, regular sausages, bologna, salami, and duck. Also, consider avoiding or limiting egg yolks and organ meats such as liver and giblets.

Foods thought to help maintain or reduce cholesterol levels include meats labeled "lean" or "extra lean" and protein-rich vegetables such as beans.[24] Limit cholesterol to less than 300 mg a day.[25]

CHAPTER 9: CONTROL YOUR PORTIONS

During the past twenty years, the portion size for many products has doubled, if not tripled.

~ U.S. Department of Health and Human Services

Portion control, along with exercise and eating the appropriate foods, is one of the key elements to living a leaner, fitter life. In this age of super-sized burgers and "all you can eat" buffets, you may find it very tempting and very easy to eat more food than you really need. But, how is one to know when enough food is enough? Do not confuse the "portion" size with the "serving" size. Recognize that a portion may contain more than one serving. A "portion" is the amount of food you choose to eat at one time, whether at home, from a box or bag, or in a restaurant. A "serving" is the amount of food listed on a product's Nutrition Facts label. The Nutrition Facts label also prominently displays the number of calories in a serving of food. The number of servings you consume determines the number of calories you actually eat.

39. BECOME FAMILIAR WITH PORTION DISTORTION

Today's food portions dwarf the food portions that the average person thought of as a serving twenty years ago. Measure one serving using some of the steps outlined in this chapter. Table 11 compares the portion sizes of selected foods today with their counterparts twenty years ago.

Table 11. Portion Distortion

Item	Portion Size Twenty Years Ago	Portion Size Today	Extra Calories
bagel	3" diameter, 140 calories	6" diameter, 350 calories	210
cheeseburger	333 calories	590 calories	257
spaghetti and meatballs	one cup spaghetti with sauce and three small meatballs, 500 calories	three cups of pasta with meat sauce and three large meatballs, 1025 calories	525
french fries	2.4 ounces, 210 calories	6.9 ounces, 610 calories	400
soda	6.5 ounces, 85 calories	20 ounces, 250 calories	165
turkey sandwich	320 calories	820 calories	500
coffee with whole milk and sugar	8 ounces, 45 calories	16 ounce mocha coffee with steamed whole milk and mocha syrup, 350 calories	305
muffin	1.5 ounces, 210 calories	4 ounces, 500 calories	290
pepperoni pizza	2 slices, 500 calories	2 large slices, 850 calories	350
chicken caesar salad	1 ½ cups, 390 calories	3 ½ cups, 790 calories	400
popcorn	5 cups, 270 calories	11 cups, 630 calories	360
cheesecake	3 ounces, 260 calories	7 ounces, 640 calories	380
chocolate chip cookie	1.5 inch diameter, 55 calories	3.5 inch diameter, 275 calories	220
chicken stir fry	2 cups, 435 calories	4 ½ cups, 865 calories	430

Source: National Heart, Lung, and Blood Institute,
U.S. Department of Health and Human Services

You would need to perform a variety of physical activities to burn off the extra calories in today's Herculean portions, such as:

- work in your garden for 35 minutes to burn off the extra calories from the larger portion of soda,
- lift weights for an hour and 30 minutes to burn off the extra cheeseburger calories, or
- clean your house for more than two and a half hours to burn off the extra calories added by the larger portion of spaghetti and meatball calories.

40. Don't Go Back For Seconds

Start with a small portion of food on your plate. Eat slowly. Wait 15 minutes and then decide whether you really need that second helping of Thanksgiving turkey. You will not regret it! It takes the brain approximately twenty minutes to realize that the stomach is full.[1] Savor your food. Just think of how much damage you can do in fifteen minutes if you do not give your brain and your stomach the opportunity to get in synch with each other.

41. Serve Your Meal on a Smaller Plate

If you find yourself tempted to put more food on the plate than you really need, try serving your meal on a smaller plate. Taking this step serves two purposes.

First, eating food from a smaller plate limits the amount of food that you can place on the plate. Secondly, the smaller plate gives the *illusion* of having more food on the plate. Think about it. What are your first thoughts when you and your friends are dining out and your meals arrive on plates that look like they are overflowing with food? You probably think, "Wow! Look at all of that food". On the contrary, when you and those same friends are dining in an upscale restaurant and the food arrives on a larger plate, i.e., you can actually see the plate, your thoughts might be somewhere along the lines of, "Hmmm. That's not much food for these prices." Yet, at the end of the evening, you are comfortably full. Perception is everything.

42. Follow the Half-Plate Rule

I ran across the half-plate rule in, of all places, a grocery store magazine.[2] The half-plate rule is simple. Look at your plate or bowl and divide it into half. Fill half of your plate with low-calorie vegetables or fruits. This now limits the amount of other items that you can place on your plate.

43. Count Your Chips

Do not eat out of the bag. Eating out of the bag, box or jar is a sure fire way to eat more than a serving of food. Use small sandwich bags and pre-portion your snacks. That way, you ensure that you have the right portion and you can make your snack choice a little healthier. Pour one serving of potato chips, nuts, or popcorn into each bag and eat that serving only. Some products such as potato chips may list the entire bag as one serving. If the snack is high in saturated fat, cut the serving size in half and bag half the recommended serving size.

44. GRAB A FIST FULL OF FOOD

"Grab a fist full of food" may sound inane, but it works. Your fist, as well as common household items[3], can help you gauge one serving size:

- One baked potato or one cup of cereal = size of a fist
- 1/2 cup of cooked rice, pasta, or potato = 1/2 baseball
- One medium fruit = a baseball
- 1/2 cup of fresh fruit = 1/2 baseball
- 1 1/2 ounces of cheese = four stacked dice
- 2 tablespoons of peanut butter = a ping pong ball
- 1/2 cup of ice cream = 1/2 baseball
- 3 ounces of meat or fish = a deck of cards or a cassette tape

PART 3

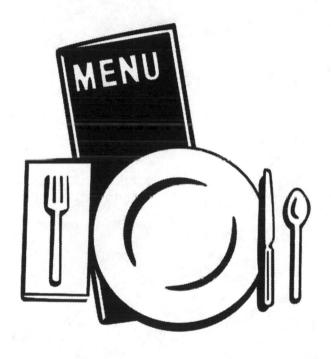

DINE SMART

CHAPTER 10: DINE RIGHT AT HOME

An estimated fifty-seven million Americans have pre-diabetes. People with pre-diabetes can prevent the development of type 2 diabetes by making changes in their diet and increasing their level of physical activity.

~ American Diabetes Association

45. BAKE, BROIL OR GRILL . . . DON'T FRY

Stay away from fried foods. The oils used to fry foods are seldom healthy and the batter used on fried foods absorbs these oils. Prepare foods in one of the following manners: steamed, broiled, baked, roasted, poached, lightly sautéed, or stir-fried.

46. STEAM YOUR VEGETABLES

Steam your fresh or frozen vegetables. Some stores now sell pre-packaged vegetables that you can steam in microwave compatible containers. Steamed vegetables retain more vitamins than boiled vegetables.

47. CUT BACK ON INSTANT OR FLAVORED MIXES

Instant and flavored mixes usually have added salt. Cook rice, pasta, and hot cereals without salt. Choose ready-to-eat breakfast cereals that are lower in sodium.

48. DON'T EAT IN FRONT OF THE TELEVISION

It is so easy to lose track of how much you are eating when you are enjoying a good television show. Your eyes and mind focus on the show while your mouth just keeps opening and closing. The same applies to going to the movies. Do you honestly think that you would enjoy drinking that icky-sweet giant soda and eating that giant tub of popcorn if you were not watching the movie?

If you must eat in front of the television or at the movies, make it a healthy, pre-portioned snack, not a major meal or junk food pig-out.

49. SPRAY AT BREAKFAST-TIME

When cooking breakfast eggs, use a non-stick pan and cooking spray. One spray of cooking spray instead of one pat of butter will save thirty-four calories.[1]

50. ADD FRUIT TO YOUR CEREAL

Put less cereal in your bowl and fill the remainder of the bowl with fruit such as bananas and berries. This translates into a full bowl and an extra dose of vitamins and minerals, and contributes to your fruit serving for the day.

51. USE PLANT-BASED OILS

Plant-based oils such as olive oil and canola oil are rich in unsaturated fats. Use olive oil-based vinaigrettes on your salads or vegetables.[2]

52. SWITCH FROM BUTTER TO SOFT TUB SPREAD

Choose a heart-healthy soft spread. Be sure to read the label to ensure that the product does not contain trans fats/partially hydrogenated oils.[3]

53. MODIFY RECIPES

Modify recipes to reduce the amount of fat and calories. For example, use light sour cream instead of eggs when making turkey meatloaf. Use part-skim ricotta cheese instead of whole-milk ricotta cheese when making lasagna. The possibilities are endless.

54. START THE DAY WITH SPINACH

Spinach, onions, and mushrooms are excellent additions to your morning omelet. Use these items in place of one of the eggs or half of the cheese in your omelet. The vegetables will give your omelet flavor and volume, with half the calories.[4]

55. EXCHANGE THE RICE OR NOODLES FOR VEGGIES

Substitute one cup of chopped vegetables for one cup of rice or noodles in your favorite dish. Use vegetables such as tomatoes, broccoli, squash, onions, or peppers.[5]

56. ADD ICE CREAM TO YOUR FRUIT

Instead of having a bowl of ice cream with a few pieces of fruit on the top, have a bowl of fruit with a teaspoon of ice cream or sorbet on top. You will save calories and get an extra dose of vitamins.

CHAPTER 11: MAKE HEALTHIER RESTAURANT CHOICES

A seemingly "healthy" turkey burger from a chain restaurant can contain as many as 890 calories and 48 grams of fat.[1]

Dining out, whether dining socially or when on the road, can present challenges. Restaurant food can be loaded with calories. When you are on the road, you may have limited dining options. By remembering a few simple tips, not only can you save money, but you can also save a lot of calories and still enjoy a good meal.

57. DON'T EMPTY THE BREADBASKET

Nibbling on the bread placed on your table while you wait for your appetizer or dinner is an easy way to add unwanted calories. Do not empty the breadbasket, no matter how hungry you may feel. If you must have a piece of bread, ask the waiter to substitute olive oil for the butter on the table.

58. SHARE AN ENTRÉE

Many restaurants, as a matter of practice, serve large entrees. Knowing this in advance, you and your dinner partner should plan ahead of time to share an entrée. Otherwise, when you arrive at the restaurant, take your time to peruse the menu. Glance at the entrees as they arrive at other tables. If the plates are overflowing with food, split an entrée with your dinner partner. Some restaurants will charge a sharing fee, but it is worth it.

59. Order Two Appetizers Instead of an Entrée

Ordering two appetizers instead of an appetizer and entrée not only saves calories, but also saves money! This choice works particularly well when dining in some Italian restaurants. Order a small salad and an appetizer portion of pasta.

60. Order a Salad with a Lean Protein

Many restaurant menus offer a choice of salads topped with lean protein. These options can provide a very satisfying meal. Top a nice selection of greens with protein such as grilled chicken or salmon. If you encounter a restaurant that does not offer this option on the menu, ask whether the chef can accommodate your special request.

61. Ask for the Salad Dressing on the Side

Once you have requested that special salad, do not spoil it with too much salad dressing. Order you salad dressing on the side. Lightly dip your fork into the dressing so that you get to taste the dressing with each bite.

Using the nutrition calculator on a popular salad bar Web site, I "built" a salad comprised of a romaine/iceberg blend with mushrooms, onions, tomatoes, Chinese noodles, cheddar cheese, and chicken. Prior to adding the salad dressing, one serving of this salad contained approximately 305 calories and 16 grams of fat. With the addition of balsamic vinaigrette, the count rises to 565 calories and 42 grams of fat![2]

62. Request a Doggie Bag

No matter what your Mom might have said to you as a child, you do not have to eat everything on your plate in one sitting. Request a doggie bag and enjoy your meal as lunch or as dinner the next day.

63. Have Your Dessert and Eat it Too

There are several ways that you can enjoy dessert and not break the calorie scale. Good desserts are the pièce de résistance of a fine meal. If there is a dessert on the menu that you really must try, share the dessert with your dinner partner. If you just do not feel like sharing, then skip the appetizer and only order an entrée so that you can enjoy the dessert. Otherwise, make a healthy choice at the end of your meal. Opt for fresh fruit as your dessert.

64. ORDER A HALF-SANDWICH

Some restaurants have half-sandwich pricing on the menu. Just as with desserts, you can enjoy the bounty but eat less of it.

65. DON'T BE TEMPTED BY BUFFETS AND SALAD BARS

All-you-can-eat buffets, including salad bars, are a bigger threat to America's health than many people realize. Have you ever taken a serious look at what is on many of these buffets?

> **Breakfast Buffet:** ham, bacon, biscuits and gravy, eggs benedict, waffles, pancakes, corned beef hash, scrapple, home fries, French toast, sausage, scrambled eggs
> **Lunch or Dinner Buffet:** barbecued spareribs, shrimp with fried rice, fried calamari, fried chicken, fried shrimp, mashed potatoes and gravy, meatloaf
> **Salad Bar:** mayonnaise-laden chicken, tuna and pasta salads, and high fat dressings such as ranch, blue cheese, and creamy Italian

If the buffet ends up as your only dining option, look for healthier choices such as green salads or lean protein such as chicken breast, sans skin.

66. THINK SMALL

On occasion, you might visit the popular fast food places. Order from the dollar menu and skip the super-size portions. In this instance, I use the term "super-size" when referring to what might be listed as the "regular" burger or fries on fast food restaurant menus. Remember the portion distortions in Chapter 9. The dollar menu typically contains portions that we once thought of as normal size servings.

Ordering from the kiddy menu is also a great alternative when dining in fast food restaurants. You can still get the fast food taste, with half the calories and fat.

67. ORDER WITH CARE IN CHAIN RESTAURANTS

Chain restaurants may be convenient and offer a lot of food for the money. But, there may be a lot more behind that "good" taste than you bargained for. The food in chain restaurants can be loaded with sodium and fat. Researchers for a nonprofit food safety and nutrition watchdog group examined the sodium content of 17 chain restaurants and found that 85 out of 102 meals had more than a day's worth of sodium.[3] According to the researchers, the top offenders were:

- Admirals' Feast with Caesar Salad, Creamy Lobster Topped Mashed Potato, Cheddar Bay Biscuit, and a Lemonade: 7,106 mg sodium
- Buffalo Chicken Fajitas (with tortillas and condiments) and a Dr Pepper: 6,916 mg sodium
- Honey-Chipotle Ribs with Mashed Potatoes with Gravy, Seasonal Vegetables, and a Dr Pepper: 6,440 mg sodium
- Tour of Italy (lasagna) with a Breadstick, Garden Fresh Salad with House Dressing, and a Coca-Cola: 6,176 mg sodium
- Chicken Parmigiana with a Breadstick, Garden Fresh Salad with House Dressing, and Raspberry Lemonade: 5,735 mg sodium

Reading this information more than piqued my interest. I decided to look up the calories and fat content of these top five offenders. The calorie and fat content listed below does not include the content of the side dishes and the beverages that accompany these items:

- Admirals' Feast (a combination of fried seafood that includes shrimp, bay scallops, clam strips and flounder) – 1,506 calories and 93.4 grams of fat[4]
- Buffalo Chicken Fajitas (crispy breaded chicken with a spicy sauce, blue cheese and applewood smoked bacon) – 1,092 calories and 77 grams of fat[5]
- Honey-Chipotle Ribs (baby back ribs with a honey-chipotle sauce) – 1,320 calories and 67 grams of fat[6]
- Tour of Italy (lasagna, chicken parmigiana and fettucine alfredo) –1,450 calories and 74 grams of fat[7]
- Chicken Parmigiana (fried parmesan-breaded chicken breasts topped with marinara sauce and mozzarella cheese) – 1,090 calories and 49 grams of fat[8]

Words and phrases to avoid when dining in chain restaurants include: glazed, battered, creamy, cream sauce, three-cheese, breaded, Alfredo, gigantic, double, fried, sweet and spicy, coated, crusted, and smothered. In simple terms, these words and phrases mean extra calories from sugar, from fats such as cheese or cream, or from frying and fat-laden breading. Look for dishes with the words charbroiled, roasted, grilled, seared, baked, or steamed.

68. MAKE HEALTHIER CHOICES WITH ETHNIC CUISINE

Take a taste adventure without compromising your new, healthier lifestyle. Select items that are lower in calories and fat. Use some of the following tips when ordering ethnic cuisine:

Chinese
Avoid battered and fried dishes, as well as dishes with MSG. Choose healthier selections such as dishes with the words steamed, jum (poached), kow (roasted), and shu (barbecued).[9]

Italian
Fettuccini Alfredo may taste good, but it's not so good on the hips and heart. The sauce contains cream, butter, and cheese. You should think red when dining Italian. Select foods prepared with red sauces, sun-dried tomatoes or crushed tomatoes. Other options include primavera (no cream), piccata (lemon), or foods that have been lightly sautéed or grilled.[10] Substitute bruschetta (bread topped with herbs and tomatoes) for garlic bread (lots of butter).

Mexican
Select items that feature spicy chicken, rice and black beans, salsa, picante, and soft tortillas.[11]

Indian
Avoid creamy curries such as korma, massala, and passanda. Choose tandoori or madras with chicken, prawns, or vegetables. Opt for plain rice and chapatti rather than pilau rice and naan.[12]

Thai
Coconut milk, which is high in saturated fat, is a major component of green and red curries. Better options are steamed or stir-fried dishes with vegetables, chicken or fish.[13]

69. MAKE MENU SUBSTITUTIONS

Scan the menu and ask the waiter whether you can combine items from one menu selection with items from another selection. For example, you might see that a lean cut of steak comes with a pasta Alfredo. You also notice that another dish on the menu comes with a side of steamed vegetables. Ask whether you can get the steamed vegetables instead of the pasta. There may be a surcharge, but the calories saved will be worth the cost.

CHAPTER 12: AVOID THE OFFICE TRAP

If you spend just $3.00 a day for breakfast and $5.00 a day for lunch, in five years you will have spent more than $10,000 buying "grab and go" meals during the workweek.

There is only one recommendation for eating at the office . . . just say "NO". For many women, the most egregious acts of self-destruction are committed during the course of the workday. Anyone who has ever worked in an office knows that someone is always baking something or bringing in donuts or celebrating with cake.

You spend more hours that are sedentary in the office than in any other place during your day. You have already eaten the bagel with cream cheese, the chips, the burger, and the candy. This afternoon is Mary's birthday celebration and you are going to help her celebrate by eating a piece of cake. Top that off with the meat loaf and mashed potatoes that you plan to eat for dinner and you will need to run several miles to burn off all of those calories. However, you are not going to run when you get home. After a long day at the office, you are going home to enjoy your meatloaf, watch some television, and go to bed so that you can get up early the next morning and begin the routine again. So, how do you avoid the office trap?

70. TAKE YOUR BREAKFAST AND LUNCH TO WORK

If you are lucky enough to have access to a refrigerator and a microwave at work, take your breakfast and lunch to work. This gives you control over the portions and calories. Pack healthy meals that include protein, grains, fruits, and vegetables.

71. Skip the Birthday Cake

The guest of honor will not be offended if you skip a slice of the homemade devil's food cake. Skip the cake and save 400 calories.[1] If you really feel guilty and feel that you must indulge, only eat one bite of the cake.

72. Say "No Thank You" to the Morning Treat

Donuts are not only loaded with calories but also contain trans fats. Skip the donuts served at the morning meeting; save some calories and keep your arteries clean. Your co-workers will understand when they start to envy that svelte body that you will soon develop.

73. Be Selective with Vending Machine Snacks

Vending machines are loaded with tempting bags and packets filled with empty calories, trans fats and sugars. A one-ounce snack pack of corn chips has the same number of calories as a small apple, one cup of whole strawberries, AND one cup of carrots with 1/4 cup of low-calorie dip combined. If you are in a pinch and find that vending machines are your only option, choose pretzels, dried fruits or trail mix.[2] Do be aware of the serving size and keep in mind the sodium/sugar content of these products.

74. Bypass the Office Candy Jar

Unless you can "eat just one", stay away from the office candy jar. Otherwise, enjoy the thigh-wreckers and prepare to move to your next dress size.

75. Save Your Money

Take the money that you save each week by packing your breakfast and lunch and open a new savings account. Call it your "vacation" account. Plan to show off your new body during your Caribbean island vacation.

PART 4

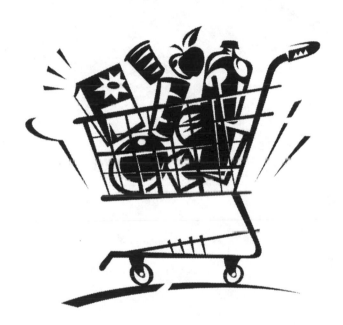

SHOP WITH A PURPOSE

CHAPTER 13: SHOP RIGHT

The Heart check mark aids you in selecting foods that meet the American Heart Association's criteria for saturated fat and cholesterol.

It is possible to eat right even while on a limited budget. How often have you purchased a bucket of fried whatever and a super-size of what is this because it was cheap and filled you? Save money and make healthy choices when you do your grocery shopping by using the next series of steps.

76. Do Not Shop When You Are Hungry

Have you ever gone into a grocery store when you were hungry and come home with items that you really did not need? Going shopping on an empty stomach can lead to impulse purchases, especially in the way of snacks.

77. Shop the Outside Aisles

The next time that you go grocery shopping, observe the layout of the store. The outside aisles contain fresh fruits, vegetables, dairy, and lean protein. In contrast, you will find the inside aisles stocked with processed foods, sugar-laden drinks, and high fat/high sodium snacks.

78. Skip the Chips and Save Money

Do you want to buy these over-priced snacks with little or no nutritional value?

One 20 oz. bag of potato chips	$4.39	2800 calories
One 8.5 oz. French onion dip	$2.99	420 calories
One 9 oz. Jalapeno/Cheddar dip	$2.99	400 calories
Two Six-packs of diet cola	$5.98	0 calories

| One 1.5 Quart Chocolate Ice Cream | $6.29 | 1680 calories |
| Price Tag | $22.64 | 5300 empty calories |

Or, would you prefer these inexpensive snacks that are loaded with vitamins and minerals?

2 lbs. of bananas	$1.58	Potassium
3 lb. bag of apples	$3.99	Potassium, Vitamin A
One 8 oz. bags celery sticks	$2.00	Potassium, Vitamin A
One 10 oz. bag (10 sticks) low-fat mozzarella	$4.59	Calcium, Protein
One 26 oz. jar all natural peanut butter	$4.79	Protein
Price Tag	$16.95	

It is possible to eat healthy and save money!

79. BUY IN SEASON

In recent years, *locally grown* has become the buzzword. That's because people are realizing that eating fresh and in season is best. Think back to your childhood. Peaches, cantaloupe and watermelon burst with flavor; corn, strawberries and blueberries were oh so sweet. When the season was over, you looked forward to eating these delicacies the next year. Buying in season ensures that you eat a variety of fruits and vegetables through the year. Buying in season also saves money since buying locally grown products may save you the costs associated with transporting food across the country.

80. STICK TO THE LIST

Always use a shopping list when you go to the grocery store. An organized approach is the best. Stick to the list and do not deviate to the inner, calorie-laden aisles. Many stores offer free food samples to entice customers to purchase new products. No matter how good the sample might taste at the time, if it is not on your list, do not buy it.

81. BUY WHOLE AND CUT YOUR OWN PORTIONS

Check the price per pound the next time that you purchase poultry. It is usually cheaper to purchase a whole chicken and cut it up yourself rather than to purchase pre-packaged chicken parts.

82. PURCHASE IN BULK

Purchase in bulk if the unit price of the smaller item is higher. The word "if" is the key in this scenario. Bigger may not always be better. Compare the unit prices to see which item gives you the most for your money. Use the information contained on the shelf labels below the product to determine the best buy.

PART 5

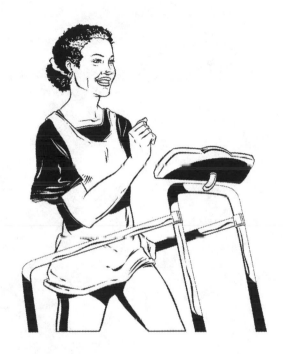

GET FIT FOR
LIFE

CHAPTER 14: BE ACTIVE

Exercising 30 minutes a day can help you lose weight, which can lower blood pressure.

~ U. S. National Library of Medicine/National Institutes of Health

Becoming and remaining physically active is vital if you want to maintain a healthy and productive life. Staying fit may help reduce risks associated with high blood pressure, diabetes and other diseases. The U.S. Department of Health and Human Services[1] found that:

- Adults 18 and older need 30 minutes of physical activity five or more days a week.
- Thirty to sixty minutes of activity broken into smaller segments of 10 or 15 minutes throughout the day has a significant health benefit.
- Moderate daily physical activity can reduce the risk of developing or dying from cardiovascular disease, type-2 diabetes, and certain cancers, such as colon cancer.
- Daily physical activity helps to lower blood pressure and cholesterol, helps prevent or retard osteoporosis, and helps reduce obesity, symptoms of anxiety and depression, and symptoms of arthritis.

Fitness activities should include all of the following types of exercise:

- Strength
- Aerobic/Endurance
- Balance
- Flexibility

Find activities that you enjoy and that are easy on your joints.

WHY BUILD MUSCLE?

A healthy body includes strong muscles and bones. Muscular strength is critical to your ability to carry out everyday activities such as household chores, carrying groceries, and lifting or moving objects. You are less likely to fall when your leg and hip muscles are strong.[2] You can strengthen your muscles using resistance training, also known as weight training. Studies have shown that lifting weights two or three times a week increases strength by building muscle mass and bone density. Strength training, especially when combined with regular aerobic exercise, can aid in reducing the signs and symptoms of numerous conditions, including arthritis, diabetes, osteoporosis, obesity, back pain, and depression.[3] Strength training[4] contributes to:

- restoration of balance
- reduction of falls
- weight maintenance
- glucose control
- a healthy state of mind
- sleep improvement
- healthy heart tissue

83. RESISTANCE TRAIN

Use dumbbells, exercise bands, or weight machines to perform resistance or strength training moves. You can also use your own body weight for strength training, such as when you do pushups. If you cannot afford a personal trainer, you can still develop a strength-training program. Consider online training programs or purchase exercise videos and fitness magazines to help you get started. Check my Web site, www.sarahalexanderfitness.com, for resources.

When traveling, check to see if the hotel has a fitness center. If a fitness center is not available, workout in your room. Take resistance bands or portable weights to aid you with your in-room workout.

CALORIES IN VERSUS CALORIES OUT: BURN FAT

The key to maintaining a healthy weight is to balance calories in with calories out. To lose weight, you should aim to burn more calories than you have taken in, i.e., increase physical activity and decrease calorie intake. Aerobic exercise is one way to burn calories. Aerobic fitness, also known as cardiovascular fitness, involves the heart, blood vessels and lungs working together to deliver oxygen-rich blood to the muscles during exercise.[5] Aerobic fitness is associated with lower risks of several diseases, including high blood pressure and coronary heart disease.[6]

84. START OUT SLOWLY

Use a sensible approach to exercise by starting out slowly if you have been inactive for a while. Begin by choosing moderate-intensity activities you enjoy the most. By choosing activities you enjoy, you will be more likely to stick with them.

85. GRADUALLY INCREASE ACTIVITY

Gradually build up the time spent doing the activity by adding a few minutes every few days or so until you can comfortably perform at least 30 minutes of per day. As the minimum amount becomes easier, gradually increase the length of time performing an activity or increase the intensity of the activity, or both.

86. VARY YOUR ACTIVITIES

Vary your activities, for both interest and the range of benefits. By constantly exploring new physical activities, you are not only challenging your body but also helping to stay interested in physical activity.

Table 8 shows the estimated number of calories women need to maintain energy levels. All three categories include the light physical activity associated with typical day-to-day life.

Table 12. Calorie Needs by Level of Physical Activity

Age (years)	Sedentary	Moderately Active	Active
31-50	1800	2000	2200
51+	1600	1800	2000-2200

Source: Dietary Guidelines for Americans, 2005

A sedentary lifestyle is one in which you only perform the light physical activity that is associated with typical day-to-day life. A moderately active woman also includes physical activity that is equivalent to walking one and one-half to three miles per day at three to four miles per hour. The lifestyle of an active woman includes physical activity equivalent to walking more than three miles per day at three to four miles per hour.

Following are some common physical activities and the calories expended per hour for each. The calorie expenditures are for a 154 person. People weighing more than 154 pounds would burn less calories and those weighing less than 154 pounds would burn more calories.[7]

Hiking	370
Light gardening/yard work	330

Dancing	330
Golf (walking and carrying clubs)	330
Bicycling <10 mph	290
Walking 3.5 mph	290
Weight lifting (light workout)	220
Stretching	110
Running/jogging (5 mph)	590
Bicycling (>10 mph)	590
Swimming (slow freestyle laps)	510
Aerobics	480
Walking (4.5 mph)	460
Heavy yard work (chopping wood)	440
Weight lifting (vigorous effort)	440
Basketball (vigorous)	440

The next time that you are tempted to eat or drink a high calorie treat, remember the following: You would need to walk more than three hours at a steady 3.5 mile per hour pace to burn off the 900 calories in the Philly cheese steak that you had for lunch.

87. TAKE THE STAIRS

Whenever possible, take the stairs rather than the elevator or escalator. Taking the stairs gets your heart pumping, burns calories, and helps to tone and firm thighs and buttocks. Make certain that you place your foot firmly on each step. You should feel the muscles in your quads, legs, and glutes, not your knees, working as your climb progresses. Remember, put safety first. Do not put yourself in an unsafe situation just for the sake of exercise.

88. EXERCISE WHILE WATCHING TV

The key to weight loss is to keep moving. You are not burning many calories by being a couch potato. Spending too many hours sitting in front of the television has been associated with increased risk of obesity and type 2 diabetes in women.[8] Researchers found that women who spent more time watching TV were more likely to smoke and drink alcohol and less likely to exercise. The study also concluded that these women also had a higher intake of saturated fats, red meat, processed meat, refined grain products, snacks, sweets/desserts, and lower intakes of fish, vegetables, fruits, and whole grains.[9] Make TV time exercise time. Perform a variety of activities, such as riding a stationary bike, walking in place, and stretching, while watching your favorite shows.

89. Exercise in the Morning

If your schedule is busy and you absolutely have no time in the evenings, exercise in the morning. Set your clock 45 minutes to an hour earlier than usual. Make exercise a priority.

90. Aim for 10,000 Steps

Make a walking goal of 10,000 steps a day. Reaching 10,000 steps is easier than you think. Buy a pedometer, do some of the following and you will easily accomplish the 10,000 steps and more.

- Get off the bus one stop early. Gradually, add on more blocks as you become more comfortable walking.
- Park your car further away from the store when you are shopping.
- Get to your local mall early and do several laps around the mall.
- Visit a zoo or museum. Both involve lots of walking while still having fun.
- Take a brisk walk after dinner.
- Take a walk around the block at lunchtime.
- Use the office printer that is located farthest away from your desk.

When walking, swing your arms while keeping your head up and your body erect. Do not swing your arms from side to side, but move them from front to back, as if you were skiing.

91. Make Walking a Tradition

Check the Internet or your local newspapers for upcoming walker events. Begin training now for walking events such as the March of Dimes, Susan G. Koman and AIDS walks. In addition, some marathons are walker friendly and you can register for either full or half-marathons. Cities such as Philadelphia, Cincinnati, Long Beach, Las Vegas, and Anchorage host walker-friendly marathons.

Balance and Stretching

Balance and stretching activities enhance your physical stability and reduce your risk of injuries. Stretching allows your body to move more freely so that you can easily accomplish everyday tasks such as tying your shoes.[4] Activities such as standing on one foot or getting up from a chair without using your hands or arms help your balance.

92. Explore the Martial Arts

T'ai Chi is a form of martial arts that involves graceful movements. You can adapt these moves for meditation or self-defense. T'ai Chi can increase both balance and flexibility. T'ai Chi may also help to lower blood pressure, and decrease stress, anxiety, and depression.[10]

93. Unwind with Yoga

Yoga can also increase balance and flexibility and help you relax too. Often referred to as hatha yoga, this discipline involves using different positions, known as poses, to stretch, relax, and strengthen the body. There are many different styles of yoga. The thing that distinguishes the yoga styles is the emphasis not the pose. Find a yoga studio that offers a variety of styles so that you can choose a style that is right for you; do not be afraid to experiment.

PART 6

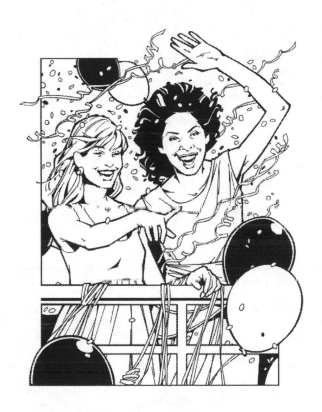

SUCCESS BEGINS WITH YOU

CHAPTER 15: NOTHING SUCCEEDS LIKE SUCCESS

I attribute my success to this—I never gave or took any excuse.

~Florence Nightingale

You have learned how to eat right and how to burn fat; now must also learn to modify your lifestyle.

94. GET SMART

Set SMART goals. SMART goals are goals that are **S**pecific, **M**easurable, **A**chievable, **R**ealistic, and **T**ime-specific. Ask yourself the following questions.

- Is my goal specific?

  "I want to lose weight" is a goal, but it is not specific. A specific goal is: "I want to lose 20 pounds by reducing calorie intake and exercising at least three times a week for the next three months."

- Is my goal measurable?

  Document your progress. For example, set a goal to weigh yourself at the end of each week and track the progress in a journal. It may help you to see it in writing. Track your progress and have concrete proof of where you were and where you are now. Also, seeing on paper that you have not exercised in five days or that you ate twice as much food as you should have eaten serves as an incentive to get moving.

- Is my goal achievable?

  "I want to lose 20 pounds by New Year's Eve" is specific, but is it achievable, particularly if New Year's Eve is only one month away? Will you give up if New

Year's Eve arrives and you can't fit into that sexy outfit that you had hoped to wear? Do not set yourself up for failure. Set a goal that is achievable, such as "I want to lose five pounds in the next 30 days". Once you have lost the first five pounds, work towards losing the next five.

- Is my goal realistic?

  "I want to run a marathon". Is this a realistic goal, especially if you have not been training and have never participated in a marathon? Although achieving this goal is not impossible, a more realistic goal may be to begin a training program and set your goal to participate in a 5K or a half-marathon.

- Is my goal time-specific?

  "I will start an exercise program" is a goal but is not time-specific? "I will exercise 30 minutes a day, three times a week, beginning on Monday" is a time-specific goal.

95. Keep a Positive Attitude

It is all about attitude. If you do not believe in yourself, who else will? There will be times when it seems like you are not making any progress or that you are actually going backwards. Sometimes, this may be the case. Be persistent. Look through your journal; what can you change? What should you add?

96. Quit Smoking

Surgeon General's warnings aside, if you continue to smoke, you defeat the purpose of eating right and exercising.

97. Limit Alcohol

Alcohol offers lots of calories, but little in the form of nutrients. Following are calorie counts for some popular alcoholic beverages. The calories listed are approximate and do not include the caloric content of your chosen mixer:

Table 13. Alcohol Calories

Beverage	Serving Size	Calories per Serving
Beer (regular)	12 oz	144
Beer (light)	12 oz	108
White wine	5 oz	100
Red Wine	5 oz	105
Sweet dessert wine	3 oz	141
80 proof distilled spirits (gin, vodka, rum, whiskey)	1.5 oz	96

Source: Dietary Guidelines 2005

98. GET A BUDDY

Surround yourself with like-minded people. Get a friend or other support person to exercise with you and join you in your healthy eating habits. Challenge your spouse or partner to a weight loss competition.

99. FORGIVE YOURSELF IF YOU SLIP

It is easy to slip back into your old ways. You might attend a party and have more food and drink than you should. View this as a temporary setback. Get back on track and keep working towards your goal.

100. DON'T MAKE EXCUSES

You can come up with a myriad of excuses as to why you did not exercise or why you did not stick to your healthy eating routine. You might say that you are too tired after work, so you no longer exercise after work. That is a lame excuse. Exercise in the morning or at lunchtime instead of in the evening. Do not let excuses destroy your progress.

101. DO IT FOR YOURSELF

Seldom does one succeed when one does something for the sake of pleasing others. You must decide that you are moving towards your new healthy lifestyle for you. Accept the praises of others; but reap the benefits of personal satisfaction when you reach your goal.

ENJOY YOUR NEW LIFE!

AFTERWORD

Eat this, not that. Drink this, not that. By now, your head must be swimming. But, it's very easy. Remember the basics:

- First, read the label.
- Eat fresh.
- Reduce sodium intake.
- Get fiber.
- Understand fats and cholesterol.
- Control portion size.
- Exercise daily.
- Build muscle.
- Make lifestyle changes.

APPENDIX A. LOW CALORIE, LOW FAT FOOD ALTERNATIVES

The following list is not intended to be exhaustive, but can be used as a guide to finding lower calorie, lower fat substitutes. In all cases, compare labels for caloric, fat, and sugar content.

Dairy, Meat, Fish and Poultry

Higher-Fat Foods	Lower-Fat Foods
DAIRY	
Evaporated whole milk	Evaporated fat-free (skim), reduced-fat (2%) milk
Whole milk	Low-fat (1%), reduced-fat (2%), fat-free milk
Ice cream	Sorbet, sherbet, low-fat or fat-free frozen yogurt
Whipping cream	Imitation whipped cream (made with fat-free milk)
Sour cream	Plain low-fat yogurt
Cream cheese	Neufchatel or "light" cream cheese or fat-free cream cheese
Cheese (cheddar, Swiss, jack)	Reduced-calorie, low-calorie or fat-free cheese
American cheese	Fat-free American or other fat-free cheese
Regular (4%) cottage cheese	Low-fat or reduced-fat cottage cheese
Whole milk mozzarella cheese	Part-skim milk, low-moisture mozzarella cheese
Whole milk ricotta cheese	Part-skim milk ricotta cheese
Coffee cream (half and half) or nondairy creamer	Low-fat or reduced-fat milk or non-fat dry powder
MEAT, FISH, AND POULTRY	
Cold-cuts, lunch meats	Low-fat cold-cuts (95 to 97% fat-free)
Hot dogs (regular)	Lower-fat hot dogs
Bacon or sausage	Canadian bacon or lean ham
Regular ground beef	Extra lean ground beef or ground turkey
Chicken or turkey with skin, duck, or goose	Chicken or turkey without skin (white meat)
Oil-packed tuna	Water-packed tuna (rinse to reduce sodium)
Beef (chuck, rib, brisket)	Beef (round, loin), trimmed of external fat
Pork (spareribs, untrimmed loin)	Pork tenderloin or trimmed, lean smoked ham
Frozen breaded fish or fried fish	Fish or shellfish, not breaded
Whole eggs	Egg whites or egg substitutes
Frozen TV dinners (containing more than 13 grams of fat per serving)	Frozen TV dinners (containing less than 13 grams of fat per serving and lower in sodium)
Chorizo sausage	Turkey sausage or vegetarian (tofu) sausage

Source: "Low-Calorie, Lower-Fat Alternative Foods", Obesity Education Initiative, National Heart, Lung and Blood Institute

Cereals, Grains, Pasta, Baked Good, Fats, Oils and Salad Dressings

Higher-Fat Foods	Lower-Fat Foods
CEREALS, GRAINS, AND PASTAS	
Ramen noodles	Rice or noodles (spaghetti, macaroni, etc.)
Pasta with white sauce (alfredo)	Pasta with red sauce (marinara)
Pasta with cheese sauce	Pasta with vegetables (primavera)
Granola	Bran flakes, crispy rice, etc.
	Cooked grits or oatmeal
BAKED GOODS	
Croissants, brioches, etc.	Hard French rolls or soft brown 'n serve rolls
Donuts, sweet rolls, muffins, scones, or pastries	English muffins, bagels, reduced-fat or fat-free muffins or scones
Party crackers	Low-fat, saltine or soda crackers (choose lower in sodium)
Cake (pound, chocolate, yellow)	Cake (angel food, white, gingerbread)
Cookies	Reduced-fat or fat-free cookies (graham crackers, ginger snaps, fig bars)
FATS, OILS AND SALAD DRESSINGS	
Regular margarine or butter	Liquid spread margarine, diet margarine, or whipped butter, tub or squeeze bottle
Regular mayonnaise	Light or diet mayonnaise or mustard
Regular salad dressings	Reduced-calorie or fat-free salad dressings, lemon juice or plain, herb flavored, or wine vinegar
Butter or margarine on toast or bread	Jelly, jam, or honey on bread or toast
Oils, shortening or lard	Nonstick cooking spray; stir-fry or sautée
	Applesauce or prune puree (as a substitute for oil or butter in baked goods)
MISCELLANEOUS	
Canned cream soups	Canned broth-based soups
Canned beans and franks	Canned baked beans with tomato sauce
Gravy (homemade with fat and/or milk)	Gravy mixes made with water or homemade with the fat skimmed off and fat-free milk
Fudge sauce	Chocolate syrup
Avocado on sandwiches	Cucumber slices or lettuce leaves
Guacamole dip or refried beans with lard	Salsa

"Low-Calorie, Lower-Fat Alternative Foods", Obesity Education Initiative
National Heart, Lung and Blood Institute

ENDNOTES

Chapter 1

1. *Statistics Related to Overweight and Obesity*, National Institute of Diabetes and Digestive and Kidney Diseases, Weight Control Information Network, win.niddk.nih.gov/statistics/#what
2. Ibid
3. *Calculate Your Body Mass Index*, U.S. Department of Health and Human Services, National Institutes of Health, www.nhlbisupport.com/bmi/bmicalc.htm
4. *How to Get to Your Healthy Weight*, Harvard School of Public Health, The Nutrition Source, www.hsph.harvard.edu/nutritionsource/healthy-weight/healthy-weight-full-story/
5. *The Health of Minority Women*, U.S. Department of Health and Human Services, Office on Women's Health, www.4woman.gov/owh/pub/minority/status.htm
6. Ibid
7. Ibid
8. *Leading Causes of Death in Females United States, 2004*, U.S. Department of Health and Human Services, Centers for Disease Control and Prevention, www.cdc.gov/Women/lcod.htm

Chapter 2

1. *How to Understand and Use the Nutrition Facts Label*, U.S. Food and Drug Administration, Center for Food Safety and Applied Nutrition, www.cfsan.fda.gov/~dms/foodlab.html
2. Ibid
3. *The Food Label*, U.S. Department of Health and Human Services, U.S. Food and Drug Administration, FDA Backgrounder, May 1999, www.cfsan.fda.gov/~dms/fdnewlab.html
4. *Food Label Helps Consumers Make Healthier Choices*, U.S. Food and Drug Administration, www.fda.gov/consumer/updates/foodlabels032708.html
5. *USDA Database for the Added Sugars Content of Selected Foods*, Nutrient Data Laboratory, Beltsville Human Nutrition Research Center (BHNRC), Agricultural Research Service

(ARS), U.S. Department of Agriculture(USDA), www.nal.usda.gov/fnic/foodcomp/Data/add_sug/addsug01.pdf

6. *Food Label Helps Consumers Make Healthier Choices*, U.S. Food and Drug Administration, www.fda.gov/consumer/updates/foodlabels032708.html

7. *The Food Label*, U.S. Department of Health and Human Services, U.S. Food and Drug Administration, FDA Backgrounder, May 1999, www.cfsan.fda.gov/~dms/fdnewlab.html

8. *Fat-Free Isn't Always "Free"*, U. S. Department of Health and Human Services, National Institutes of Health, National Heart Lung and Blood Institute, www.nhlbi.nih.gov/health/public/heart/obesity/wecan/learn-it/fat-free.htm

9. *Product Info & Recipes*, Herr Foods, Inc., www.herrs.com/Products/Products.html

10. *The Food Label*, U.S. Department of Health and Human Services, U.S. Food and Drug Administration, FDA Backgrounder, May 1999, www.cfsan.fda.gov/~dms/fdnewlab.html

11. Ibid

12. *Food Label Helps Consumers Make Healthier Choices*, U.S. Food and Drug Administration, www.fda.gov/consumer/updates/foodlabels032708.html

13. Ibid

14. *Product Info & Recipes*, Herr Foods, Inc., www.herrs.com/Products/Products.html

15. *National Organic Program: Organic Production and Handling Standards*, U.S. Department of Agriculture, Agricultural Marketing Service, www.ams.usda.gov

16. Ibid

17. *Shoppers Guide*, The Environmental Working Group, www.foodnews.org

18. *The Food Label*, U.S. Department of Health and Human Services, U.S. Food and Drug Administration, FDA Backgrounder, May 1999, www.cfsan.fda.gov/~dms/fdnewlab.html

19. Ibid

20. *Dietary Guidelines for Americans 2005*, U.S. Department of Health and Human Services/U.S. Department of Agriculture, www.health.gov/dietaryguidelines/dga2005/document/pdf/DGA2005.pdf

21. Ibid

Chapter 3

1. *Don't Forget Breakfast*, Prevention.com, Rodale, Inc., www.prevention.com/cda/article/don%20t-forget-breakfast/

2. *McDonald's USA - Food, Nutrition, & Fitness*, www.mcdonalds.com/usa/eat.html

3. *starbucksÒ beverages*, Starbucks Corporation, www.starbucks.com/retail/nutrition_beverage_detail.asp

4. *starbucksÒ food*, Starbucks Corporation, www.starbucks.com/retail/nutrition_food_detail.asp

5. Ibid

6. *How to Understand and Use the Nutrition Facts Label*, U.S. Food and Drug Administration, Center for Food Safety and Applied Nutrition, www.cfsan.fda.gov/~dms/foodlab.html

7. *Philly's Favorite Foods: Cheese steak and Cheese Fries, The Meal That Made Philadelphia Famous*, Analysis by: Lauren Hudson, MS, RD, Candace Cantwell, RD, Marianne Petrella, RD and Olga Antonopoulos, last updated: 6/14/2000, The University of Pennsylvania Health System, www.pennhealth.com/health_info/nutrition/philly/chstk.html

8. *How to Understand and Use the Nutrition Facts Label*, U.S. Food and Drug Administration, Center for Food Safety and Applied Nutrition, www.cfsan.fda.gov/~dms/foodlab.html

9. Ibid

10. *Is Eight Enough? U Researcher Says Drink Up and Tells Why*, The University of Utah, University Healthcare, www.healthcare.utah.edu/publicaffairs/news/archive/2003/news_74.html

11. *Water: How much should you drink every day?*, MayoClinic.com, Mayo Foundation for Medical Education and Research, www.mayoclinic.com/health/water/NU00283

12. *Pepsi Product Information*, Pepsico, Inc., www.pepsiproductfacts.com

13. *New Analysis Suggests Diet Soda Paradox; Less Sugar, More Weight*, HSC News, June 14, 2005, Volume XXXVIII, Issue 24, University of Texas Health Science Center at San Antonio, www.uthscsa.edu/HSCnews/singleformat.asp?newID=1539&SearchID=.

14. *Vitamin Water*, Glacéau, www.vitaminwater.com

15. *Protein: Moving Closer to Center Stage*, The Nutrition Source, Harvard School of Public Health, www.hsph.harvard.edu/nutritionsource/what-should-you-eat/protein-full-story/index.html

16. *Protein in Diet*, Medline Plus Medical Encyclopedia, National Institutes of Health/ Department of Health & Human Services, U.S. National Library of Medicine, www.nlm.nih.gov/medlineplus/ency/article

17. Ibid

18. Ibid

Chapter 4

1. *How to Use Fruits and Vegetables to Management Your Weight*, Centers for Disease Control, www.cdc.gov/nccdphp/dnpa/healthyweight/healthy_eating/fruits_vegetables.htm

2. Ibid

3. *Fruit & Vegetable Benefits: Nutrient Information*, Centers for Disease Control and Prevention, www.fruitsandveggiesmatter.gov/benefits/nutrient_guide.html

4. Ibid

5. Ibid

6. Ibid

7. *How Much Fruit is Needed Daily*, Inside the Pyramid, U.S. Department of Agriculture, MyPyramid.gov, www.mypyramid.gov/pyramid/fruits_amount.aspx#

8. *Fruit & Vegetable Benefits: Nutrient Information*, Centers for Disease Control and Prevention, www.fruitsandveggiesmatter.gov/benefits/nutrient_guide.html

9. *Why is it Important to Eat Vegetables?*, Inside the Pyramid, U.S. Department of Agriculture, MyPyramid.gov, www.mypyramid.gov/pyramid/vegetables_why.html

10. Ibid

11. *What Foods are in the Vegetable Group?*, Inside the Pyramid, U.S. Department of Agriculture, MyPyramid.gov, www.mypyramid.gov/pyramid/vegetables.html

12. *Fruit & Vegetable Benefits: Nutrient Information*, Centers for Disease Control and Prevention, www.fruitsandveggiesmatter.gov/benefits/nutrient_guide.html

13. Ibid

14. Ibid

15. *How to Use Fruits and Vegetables to Management Your Weight*, Centers for Disease Control, www.cdc.gov/nccdphp/dnpa/healthyweight/healthy_eating/fruits_vegetables.htm

Chapter 5

1. *What You Should Know About Calcium*, National Osteoporosis Foundation, www.nof.org/prevention/calcium2.htm

2. Ibid

3. Ibid

4. Ibid

5. *Nutrition Labels Show You Where to Find Calcium*, Calcium Education Program Leader's Guide, U.S. Food and Drug Administration, Center for Food Safety and Applied Nutrition, www.cfsan.fda.gov/~dms/ca-2.html

6. *Thinking About Calcium? Find It In Food First*, National Dairy Council, www.nebmilk.org/HP/handouts/ThinkingCalcium.pdf

Chapter 6

1. *Sodium Health Article*, Greg Annussek, Rebecca J. Frey PhD, The Gale Group Inc., Gale, Detroit, Gale Encyclopedia of Alternative Medicine, 2005, www.healthline.com/galecontent/sodium/2

2. *Reduce Salt and Sodium in Your Diet*, National Heart, Lung, and Blood Institute, National Institutes of Health, www.nhlbi.nih.gov/hbp/prevent/sodium/flavor.htm

3. *Dietary Guidelines for Americans 2005*, U.S. Department of Health and Human Services/ U.S. Department of Agriculture, www.health.gov/dietaryguidelines/dga2005/document/pdf/DGA2005.pdf

4. *Shake the Salt Habit*, American Heart Association, americanheart.org/presenter.jhtml?identifier=2106

5. *Flavor That Food, Your Guide to Lowering High Blood Pressure*, National Heart, Lung, and Blood Institute, National Institutes of Health, www.nhlbi.nih.gov/hbp/prevent/sodium/flavor.htm

6. Ibid

Chapter 7

1. *Most Frequently Asked Questions About Sports Nutrition*, The President's Council on Physical Fitness, www.fitness.gov/publications/council/faq_pdf.pdf

2. *Carbohydrates*, Medline Plus, U. S. National Library of Medicine and the National Institutes of Health, www.nlm.nih.gov/medlineplus/carbohydrates.html

3. Ibid

4. Ibid

5. *What Foods are in the Grain Group?*, Inside the Pyramid, U. S. Department of Agriculture, www.mypyramid.gov/pyramid/grains.html

6. Ibid

7. Ibid

8. Ibid

9. Ibid

10. *What Foods are in the Grain Group?*, Inside the Pyramid, U. S. Department of Agriculture, www.mypyramid.gov/pyramid/grains.html

11. Ibid

Chapter 8

1. *Nutrition Facts*, American Heart Association, www.americanheart.org

2. *Specific Types of Fat*, Nutrition & Recipes, American Diabetes Association, www.diabetes.org/nutrition-and-recipes/nutrition/foodlabel/specific-fats.jsp

3. *Trans Fats*, American Heart Association, www.americanheart.org

4. Ibid

5. *Specific Types of Fat*, Nutrition & Recipes, American Diabetes Association, www.diabetes.org/nutrition-and-recipes/nutrition/foodlabel/specific-fats.jsp

6. Ibid

7. Ibid

8. Ibid

9. *Consumer FAQ - 'Better' Fats (Monounsaturated and Polyunsaturated Fats)*, American Heart Association, www.americanheart.org/presenter.jhtml?identifier=3046644#def_omega_3

10. *Tip Sheet: Fats and Oils to Choose, How You Can Lower Your Cholesterol Levels*, National Heart Lung and Blood Institute, http://nhlbisupport.com/chd1/Tipsheets/tipsheet-satfat.htm

11. *What You Need to Know About Mercury in Fish and Shellfish*, Backgrounder for the 2004 FDA/EPA Consumer Advisory, U. S. Food and Drug Administration, www.fda.gov/oc/opacom/hottopics/mercury/backgrounder.html

12. Ibid

13. Ibid

14. *The Salmon Scam: 'Wild' Often Isn't*, ConsumerReports.org, www.consumerreports.org/cro/food/food-shopping/meats-fish-protein-foods/mislabeled-salmon/salmon-8-06/overview/0608_salmon_ov.htm

15. *Calories: Know Your Numbers*, American Association for Retired People, www.aarp.org/health/healthyliving/articles/calories_know_your_numbers.html

16. *Consumer FAQ - 'Better' Fats (Monounsaturated and Polyunsaturated Fats)*, American Heart Association, www.americanheart.org

17.Ibid

18. *What is Cholesterol*, American Heart Association, www.americanheart.org/presenter.jhtml?identifier=3046103

19. *The Two Sources of Cholesterol*, American Heart Association, www.americanheart.org/presenter.jhtml?identifier=3046105

20. *LDL and HDL Cholesterol: What's Bad and What's Good?*, American Heart Association, http://www.americanheart.org/presenter.jhtml?identifier=180

21. *Why is it important to make lean or low-fat choices from the Meat and Beans group?*, Inside the Pyramid, http://www.mypyramid.gov/pyramid/meat_why_print.html

22. Ibid

23. Ibid

24. Ibid

25. *Reading Food Labels*, American Heart Association, www.americanheart.org

Chapter 9

1. *Nutri-Facts Issue #3*, Texas Cooperative Extension, fcs.tamu.edu/food_and_nutrition/nutrifacts/issue3.pdf

2. *Watching Portions Can Be Easy With the Half-Plate Rule*, Jane Andrews, Corporate Nutrition Manager, Wegman's Menu Magazine, Summer 2008, page 79

3. *Just Enough for You: About Food Portions*, Weight-control Information Network, National Institutes of Health, U.S. Departme;nt of Health and Human Services, win.niddk.nih.gov/publications/just_enough.htm#difference

Chapter 10

1. *Cutting Calories,* Healthy Weight - it's not a diet, it's a lifestyle!, Centers for Disease Control and Prevention, www.cdc.gov/nccdphp/dnpa/healthyweight/healthy_eating/cutting_calories.htm
2. *The Bottom Line: Choose healthy fats, limit saturated fat, and avoid trans fat,* The Nutrition Source: Fats and Cholesterol, Harvard School of Public Health, www.hsph.harvard.edu/nutritionsource/what-should-you-eat/fats-and-cholesterol/index.html
3. Ibid
4. *How to Use Fruits and Vegetables to Help Manage Your Weight,* Healthy Weight - it's not a diet, it's a lifestyle!, Centers for Disease Control and Prevention, www.cdc.gov/healthyweight/healthy_eating/fruits_vegetables.html
5. Ibid

Chapter 11

1. *Ruby Tuesday Menu Guide, May 2009,* Ruby Tuesday, Inc., www.rubytuesday.com/files/allergen.pdf
2. *Calculator,* Saladworks, www.saladworks.com
3. *"Heart Attack Entrees with Side Orders of Stroke",* Newsroom, News from CSPI, Center for Science in the Public Interest, cspinet.org/new/200905111.html
4. *Nutrition Facts,* Red Lobster, www.redlobster.com/health/nutrition/dinner.asp
5. *Nutritional Information,* Chili's, www.brinker.com/gr/nutritional/chilis_nutrition_menu.pdf
6. Ibid
7. *Nutritional Information,* Darden Concepts Inc., www.olivegarden.com/menus/garden_fare/nutrition_information.asp
8. Ibid
9. *Eating Healthy with Ethnic Food,* National Heart, Lung and Blood Institute, www.nhlbi.nih.gov/health/public/heart/obesity/lose_wt/eth_dine.htm
10. Ibid
11. Ibid
12. *Making Healthier Choices,* Food Standards Agency, www.eatwell.gov.uk/healthydiet/eatingouthealthily/healthierchoices/
13. Ibid

Chapter 12

1. *What's in the Food You Eat?*, Agricultural Research Service, U.S. Department of Agriculture, http://www.ars.usda.gov/Services/docs.htm?docid=17032
2. *How to Use Fruits and Vegetables to Help Manage Your Weight*, Healthy Weight - it's not a diet, it's a lifestyle!, Centers for Disease Control and Prevention, www.cdc.gov/healthyweight/healthy_eating/fruits_vegetables.html

Chapter 14

1. *Physical Activity Facts*, The President's Council on Physical Fitness and Sports, U.S. Department of Health and Human Services, fitness.gov/resources/facts/index.html
2. *Exercise and Physical Activity: Getting Fit for Life,* National Institute on Aging, U.S. National Institutes of Health, www.nia.nih.gov/HealthInformation/Publications/exercise.htm
3. *Grow Stronger - Strength Training for Older Adults*, Centers for Disease Control and Prevention, www.cdc.gov/nccdphp/dnpa/physical/growing_stronger/why.htm
4. Ibid
5. *Adult Fitness Test*, The President's Council on Physical Fitness and Sports, U.S. Department of Health and Human Services, www.adultfitnesstest.org
6. Ibid
7. *Dietary Guidelines for Americans 2005*, U.S. Department of Health and Human Services/ U.S. Department of Agriculture, www.health.gov/dietaryguidelines/dga2005/document/pdf/DGA2005.pdf
8. *Television Watching and Other Sedentary Behaviors in Relation to Risk of Obesity and Type 2 Diabetes Mellitus in Women,* Frank B. Hu, MD, PhD; Tricia Y. Li, MD; Graham A. Colditz, MD, DrPH; Walter C. Willett, MD, DrPH; JoAnn E. Manson, MD, DrPH , *JAMA.* 2003;289:1785-1791., Journal of the American Medical Association, jama.ama-assn.org
9. Ibid
10. *Stay Young with Tai Chi,* Caroline Bollinger, www.prevention.com/cda/article/stay-young-with-tai-chi

Printed in the United States
by Baker & Taylor Publisher Services